T0385640

# Remaking the Urban Social Contract

**THE URBAN AGENDA**

Series Editor, Michael A. Pagano

*A list of books in the series appears at the end of this book.*

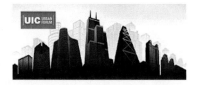

# Remaking the Urban Social Contract

## Health, Energy, and the Environment

EDITED BY MICHAEL A. PAGANO

University of Illinois at Chicago

PUBLISHED FOR THE
COLLEGE OF URBAN PLANNING
AND PUBLIC AFFAIRS (CUPPA),
UNIVERSITY OF ILLINOIS AT CHICAGO,
BY THE UNIVERSITY OF ILLINOIS PRESS
Urbana, Chicago, and Springfield

The College of Urban Planning and Public Affairs of the University of Illinois at Chicago and the University of Illinois Press gratefully acknowledge that publication of this book was assisted by a grant from the John D. and Catherine T. MacArthur Foundation.

Printed and bound in Great Britain by
Marston Book Services Ltd, Oxfordshire

Library of Congress Control Number: 2016942752
ISBN 978-0-252-04069-6 (hardcover)
ISBN 978-0-252-08220-7 (paperback)
ISBN 978-0-252-09913-7 (e-book)

# Contents

# Preface and Acknowledgments

The political mood of the United States in the early twenty-first century has been characterized as polarizing. A 2014 poll by the Pew Research Center found that the typical median Republican "is now more conservative than 94% of Democrats, compared with 70% twenty years ago. And the median Democrat is more liberal than 92% of Republicans, up from 64%" (see "7 Things to Know about Polarization in America," June 12, 2014, www. pewresearch.org). Polarizing views can bring change in policies, programs and rules. And polarizing views can manifest themselves in challenges to the status quo, including the social contract that binds together people and communities.

The politically tumultuous 1960s and early 1970s in the United States resulted in national, state, and local governments promulgating policies designed to address a host of societal issues, including a degrading environment (e.g., the National Environmental Policy Act of 1969), unaffordable health care for the poor and elderly (e.g., Medicaid and Medicare in 1965), and energy conservation (e.g., fuel efficiency standards in 1975). Although a broad commitment to meet these societal issues created a broad social contract among the people, the contract is becoming unraveled and contested even as important advances in these three areas have been undertaken in the past decade. The challenges to the old social compact are most visibly played out in the nation's metropolitan regions, which generate 85 percent of the gross domestic product. Attacks on government regulation of health, energy, and environment issues coupled with the recent contraction of the economy and challenges to the validity of scientific inquiry have created a political situation in which metropolitan regions and cities are grappling again with redefining, revising, and remaking the social contract that prevailed for nearly half a century. With particular emphasis on the social contracts and political agreements on health, energy, and environmental policies of the last forty to fifty years, the 2015 UIC Urban Forum focuses on the substantive and philosophical shifts in the urban social contract and examines the remaking of urban social contracts today.

The 2015 event was cochaired by Cook County Board president Toni Preckwinkle, president and CEO of the Chicago Community Trust (CCT) Terry Mazany, and UIC chancellor Michael Amiridis. The daylong event was held September 17, 2015, beginning with two morning panels moderated by WBEZ news reporters. The four afternoon panels were organized around the themes of the four white papers. The day's events ended with a discussion on engaging communities and neighborhoods in conversations to spark meaningful dialogue and build authentic relationships for a more just and democratic society. Mazany, who spearheaded citywide On the Table events in 2014 and 2015 for the express purpose of bringing people together to explore what can be done to make the city a better place, discussed community building with Joseph Hoereth, who directs UIC's Institute for Policy and Civic Engagement (IPCE). Mazany and Hoereth ended the day's conversation by inviting proposals from the audience to design and implement a targeted project that would facilitate building communities around a social contract to be funded by CCT and IPCE. The conference ended by encouraging creative solutions to challenging problems that would build healthy, sustainable, and vibrant environments.

The 2015 UIC Urban Forum was organized by an executive committee that chose the theme of the conference, a committee of UIC scholars that identified the white papers and the authors, an external advisory board that recommended participants for the morning panels, and an operations committee responsible for organizing and planning the conference. The executive committee, which I chaired, included the UIC Great Cities Institute director Teresa Córdova, and the associate chancellor for Government and Public Affairs, Michael Redding. The UIC Committee of Academic Advisors included George Crabtree, Constance Miles Dallas, Dennis Judd, Cynthia Klein-Banai, Elizabeth Kocs, David Perry, Jesus Ramirez-Valles, and Steve Schlickman.

The external board of advisors includes the following:

- Clarence Anthony, executive director, National League of Cities
- MarySue Barrett, president, Metropolitan Planning Council
- Henry Cisneros, former secretary, HUD; former mayor, San Antonio; founder and chairman, CityView
- Michael Coleman, mayor, Columbus
- Rahm Emanuel, mayor, Chicago

- Lee Fisher, president and CEO, CEOs for Cities
- Karen Freeman-Wilson, mayor, Gary
- Bruce Katz, director of the Metropolitan Policy Program, Brookings Institution
- Jeff Malehorn, president and CEO, World Business Chicago
- Terry Mazany, president and CEO, Chicago Community Trust
- Toni Preckwinkle, president, Cook County Board
- Joseph Szabo, executive director, Chicago Metropolitan Agency for Planning
- Susana Vasquez, executive director, LISC Chicago

Participants on the panels included the following:

- John Lumpkin, senior vice president, Robert Wood Johnson Foundation
- LaMar Hasbrouck, executive director, National Association of County and City Health Organizations
- John Jay Shannon, CEO, Cook County Health System
- Natalie Moore, WBEZ
- Henry Henderson, director, National Resources Defense Council, Midwest
- David Ullrich, executive director, Great Lakes and St. Lawrence Cities Initiative
- Suzanne Malec-McKenna, executive director, Chicago Wilderness
- Shannon Heffernan, WBEZ
- William Kling, School of Public Health, University of Illinois at Chicago
- Emily Stiehl, School of Public Health, University of Illinois at Chicago
- Norbert Riedel, president and CEO, Naurex
- Terry Vanden Hoek, chair of Emergency Medicine, University of Illinois at Chicago
- Julie Morita, commissioner, Chicago Department of Public Health
- Anthony Townsend, research director, Institute for the Future
- Moira Zellner, Department of Urban Planning and Policy, University of Illinois at Chicago
- John Edel, CEO, the Plant
- Elizabeth Kocs, the Energy Initiative, University of Illinois at Chicago
- Howard Learner, president and executive director, Environmental Law and Policy Center
- Cynthia Klein-Banai, associate chancellor for sustainability, University of Illinois at Chicago

- John Flavin, executive director, Chicago Innovation Exchange
- David McDonald, Global Development Studies, Queen's University
- Dennis Judd, Department of Political Science, University of Illinois at Chicago
- Heather Alderman, president, Illinois Children's Healthcare Foundation
- Peter Skosey, executive vice president, Metropolitan Planning Council

More than five hundred attendees listened, learned, and participated in the ongoing debate on what constitutes the urban social contract in the contemporary period and what they can do as individuals and communities in creating a better, just, and resilient city. The 2015 UIC Urban Forum was designed to facilitate such a conversation and change.

The success of the 2015 Urban Forum is in no small respect due to the dedication of the core staff who invested untold hours in planning, designing, and managing the event. In particular, I am indebted to the outstanding conference management skills of Jenny Sweeney and Cybele Abrams, who orchestrated the event with the generous support of Jasculca-Terman Associates, especially Karla Bailey. Other UIC personnel who were active and supportive of the various tasks and activities of the process include Jennifer Woodard, Darcy Evon, Norma Ramos, Bill Burton, Megan Houston, Kristin Unger, and Rona Heifetz. I am deeply grateful to the entire team for their superb job in creating the event and for their indomitable spirit of working together for a successful event.

The editorial assistance and manuscript supervision by Megan Houston, who was responsible for writing the summary of the panelists' conversations (part 3 of this book, which synthesizes the salient comments from the panelists) and who with Rudy Faust were responsible for the book production process, are owed a deep debt of gratitude.

The annual UIC Urban Forum offers thought-provoking, engaged, and insightful conferences on critical urban issues in a venue to which all of the world's citizens are invited.

Michael A. Pagano
Director of the UIC Urban Forum
Dean, College of Urban Planning and Public Affairs, University of Illinois
at Chicago
January 2016

# PART ONE
# OVERVIEW

# The Social Contract

## *A Political and Economic Overview*

DAVID C. PERRY AND
NATALIA VILLAMIZAR-DUARTE
UNIVERSITY OF ILLINOIS AT CHICAGO

From its origin, the notion of a social contract seems to be related to differ-ent features of the collective, sometimes based on society and other times based on specific institutions. From Socrates's argument about the need to obey human law to ensure the organization and functioning of society to a critical contemporary understanding of social rules as possible instruments of social control, theories about the social contract have historically accom-panied the philosophical and political debate about the role of the state and the making of public policy. This chapter suggests that the contemporary shift in the balance of political and economic power represents an opportunity to review social contract theories from various understandings of the changing role of the state and the rise of economic power.

## INTRODUCTION

From its origins, the notion of the social contract seems to be related to dif-ferent features of the collective, sometimes based on society and sometimes based on specific institutions. Critiques of the monarchy are often based on the lack of a social contract: some individuals get to be the government, and governmental power is granted by an external influence (God) that cannot be contested. Society is framed by the monarch. The problem is that, as John Locke would later argue, there are rights that each individual has and those rights, collectively, amount to a society that is larger than the monarch. Thus, the notion of the social contract is embedded in each individual, but the nature of the social contract is collective (i.e., social) not individual. The social contract is viewed, therefore, as a collective enterprise and as a relational or social entity; in turn, society is a collective that requires things that are foundational and structural: that is, public goods and the means (regulations) to ensure access to them. These foundations, embedded in the social contract, are the responsibility of the government (the sovereign). But both liberal and now new or neoliberal approaches have, successively, pared down the collective nature of government, making even the foundations of government more individual in their basic rights. Does this process of devolution to the private management of public affairs resemble the social contract under the unique rule of the monarch?

From Socrates's argument on the need to obey human law to ensure the organization and functioning of society to critical contemporary understandings of social rules as possible instruments of social control, theories about the social contract have historically accompanied the philosophical and political debate about states and, more broadly, about the government of societies.[1] Questions about the contractual nature of the relations between individuals and societies have been raised since ancient times. This contractual nature assumes both a moral bond between persons to act within the frameworks of the society in which they live and, more recently, a political obligation of the society to ensure the maintenance of such frameworks.

Thomas Hobbes, John Locke, Jean-Jacques Rousseau, and other early proponents of modern social contract theories extended their own theoretical arguments for a social contract from a critique of monarchies to various conceptualizations of human nature that could transform the government of societies. More contemporary theorists, such as John Rawls and David Gauthier, proposed an understanding of the social contract where the relational moral frameworks were informed by self-awareness and recognition of the other rather than by external enforcements from the society through the sovereign. More recent theories have faced criticism from more critical perspectives that question the nature of the relations of power and the greater role of the social contract in the legitimation of power as a tool of social control. Even more, these approaches have pointed out the existence of multiple manifestations of the social contract regarding roles, positions, and power relations in society.

These longstanding examinations have been informed by and in turn have widely informed political debates about the role of both individuals and governments in the development of societies. However, the contemporary shift in the balance of political and economic power give us the opportunity to review social contract theories from an understanding of the changing role of the supportive state in the era of rising market or economic power. In this changing political-economic context, it appears to be important to explore what the social contract looks like today. What sort of shape is the social contract in? Are we facing a need to resurrect the social contract and, if so, in whose interests? Is it the "collective version" elaborated by Rousseau, or the "private version" presented by Locke, or the "individual version" advocated by Rawls and Gauthier, or something else altogether that provides a new "collective understanding" of urban living?

## THE RISE OF THE MODERN SOCIAL CONTRACT

The questioning of monarchies as adequate systems of government and consolidations into nation-states drives various theoretical constructions of the narrative of the social contract. In considering what entails a "social contract," we can begin with the formal relationships between a defined region's people in the production of a type of society that would be embedded in the notion of a "state."

### Hobbes, Locke, Rousseau, and Smith on the Sovereign

Hobbes, Locke, and Rousseau all proposed theories of the social contract that offered critiques of the unquestionable power of the sovereign (the monarch). Hobbes's understanding of the social contract arose from his studies on human nature that, in turn, informed his notions of morality and politics. His critiques were directed at the nature of sovereign power, either the "divine power" of the king that linked political obligation to religious obligation or the "parliamentary power" that linked political obligation to society. Contrariwise, he proposed that obligations should be based on individual choice. But individuals will, by choice, yield power to the sovereign in order to ensure the continued existence of society.

Hobbes also argues that social outcomes, even when they seem to be detached from people, are the result of individual behavior. Actions, he claims, are choices that depend on the interactions between individuals that will create a chain of cause and effect. In this sense, society is constructed by mechanical responses to the stimuli of the world that seem to be more a reaction than a rational action. However, Hobbes argues, these subjective choices are moral and thus, they are the reflection of individual preferences, the expression of what every individual believed to be in his or her best interests according to each individual's moral standards, beliefs, and desires.

Therefore, the pursuit of self-interest is rational, since it is a choice to maximize and make efficient the pursuit of such ends.[2]

In this sense, Hobbes argues, therefore, that "rationality" is instrumental and it is why individuals, acting "rationally," will submit to a higher political authority. By choosing to submit to a higher authority, individuals maximize their self-interest by agreeing to a "social contract" that allows people to live together without fear of death (offering them security) and with guaranteed efficiency (development). In this way, Hobbes's arguments provide two key elements to a theory of the social contract: the recognition of equal rights and common laws; and the need for enforcement mechanisms embedded in the figure of a sovereign to which individuals agree to yield this power. The social contract, Hobbes argues, is the very basis of society—it is the individual's agreement to live collectively under an authority, which is the only possible way to ensure the maximization of self-interest collectively. And no matter how poorly implemented or biased the management of the state can become, the state is the *only* institution that can ensure order. Since Hobbes, most social contract theory has promoted the status quo and a hierarchical division of power. The maintenance of structures or institutions is presented, according to Hobbes, as a foundational pillar of society and means that every challenge to these structures will be condemned for putting at risk the only institution that can prevent us from the fearful state of nature.

Hobbes's social contract is formulated from the opposition of interest and passions. It is an attempt to operationalize a countervailing strategy to define which passion becomes the "tamer" of the others.[3] By presenting passions as the drivers of human actions, the reflections of individual preferences, he introduces the notion of self-interest as part of the human nature. In addition to being self-interested, or maybe because of this self-interest, humans are also rational and therefore, for Hobbes, reason is mainly instrumental in fulfilling one's own passions. The advantage of a world governed by such interest is framed in its predictability since the pursuit of self-interested individuals will be expected to be methodical. This belief is based on the assumption of a *uniform* human nature, where everyone's self-interest is essentially the same and thus self-interest can be translated into a collective or public interest where its pursuit will be predictable, so that the others will know what to expect and how to produce the possibility of mutual gain. Thus, Hobbes provides a theory of the social contract that is the result of the countervailing strategy that mediates between passions and reason. For Hobbes, sovereign power derives from the ability to assume this mediating role and consequently the collective good will be "the by-product of individuals acting predictably in accordance with their economic interest."[4]

Locke's approach to the social contract also reviews the relationship between individuals and authority but does so quite differently. Locke's state of nature has mechanisms of self-control and thus discloses a perfect liberty that exists in this state of nature. However, even with such a notion of "perfect liberty," Locke argues that this does not necessarily mean a lack of moral values. The state of nature for Locke is pre-political but not without laws that bound the *relational* human condition. These laws of nature are given by God, which means *all* people have equal opportunities to pursue their self-interest but they are bound to respect all others who are equal in their pursuits. People are free only in how they find one another—which means they are bound to not harm one another. Locke's pre-political state of nature is, therefore, not a state of war. It can only become one when there is a dispute over property, and there is no other way to solve such a dispute since the state of nature lacks civil authority. This problem of unresolved dispute is the key reason why people will agree to create civil government and consequently leave the state of nature.

It is in this argument that Locke introduces "property" as a key component of the relationships between individuals. Private property has a collective dimension, since it is only through the act of communication and subsequent "consent of all mankind to make [the commons] his" that this occurs.[5] With this, Locke proposes an instrumental notion where property produces a collective understanding, and hence he transforms the social contract. Private property originates in the labor put into things by people and it is, therefore, the origin of collective relationships. Labor over things is, at the same time, a right and an obligation, says Locke. It is through labor that private property is claimed and communicated to the rest of society. Since all people begin as equal in God's eyes, then every person is entitled to the share of nature that he or she creates in the property he or she builds through his or her own labor. Thus, the protection of private (through an individual's labor) property and the ensuring of its proper use become key elements of Locke's theory of social contract and a basis of civic government.

Thus Locke's concern for civil government leads him to create a narrative in which property becomes the central instrument with which to frame the system of symbols that determine collective interactions, recognition, acceptance, and consent. However, this law of man needs to be rooted in something higher that he defines, as previously discussed, as the state of nature that, as we said, is a state of perfect freedom for individual human action that is bounded only by the law of nature. However, the law of nature, for Locke, is relational. It depends on others, and it requires an understanding of how individual freedom affects others. Locke's argument assumes a natural unevenness in society. In this fashion, pluralism is founded in difference, and Locke sees class relations as natural.

By collectively agreeing to the need to establish frames (or laws) for individual relations, people become subject to the public interest and, therefore, to the will of the majority. With this agreement, people gain a political system of law that will ensure the fulfillment of the social contract between individuals and institutions with the necessary power to enforce laws. Locke's justification of this political system is the protection of property and well-being. And people have the right to defy and resist authority when the socially created civic sovereign does not fulfill its part of the social contract. Therefore, Locke's relational view of the social contract entails both conformity and contestation.

Rousseau's notion of the social contract is based on the expansion of society, collectively, but it is also understood in terms of individual rights and needs. For Rousseau, the notion of the social contract lies in each individual having a *collective* identity. For him, the role of government is to secure and otherwise maintain that identity. The social contract is, therefore, a social construction, a form of social organization in which the role of the state is to assure and guarantee rights, liberties or freedoms, and equality. The division of labor, time for leisure, and property constitute mechanisms found in the state of nature, which turn into elements of judgment and competition and thus can become instruments of inequality. The state and its laws should be products of the general will of the people through which individual natural rights are transformed into civic liberties (freedom of speech, equality, assembly, etc.) Rousseau argued that people, therefore, are born *free* to follow the rules of society.

In Rousseau's view, the state existed to protect the natural rights of the citizens and when government failed in such protection, citizens, as the source of the state, have the right to intervene themselves. He proposed, therefore, a key difference between state and government: the government can be overruled but the state cannot, since the latter is the civil basis of the social contract. He proposed a dynamic theory of the social contract whereby people moved from a state of nature to a modern society, therefore shifting from a naturalized social contract to a normative one. The first stage of this dynamic transformation is one of the individual and his or her self-interest of nature while the second stage is the move to the collective action with which to balance competition and inequality. In this latter stage of such theorization, comparison between people is developed in public values and standards.

In this approach, private property is an element that introduces inequality and leads to the development of social classes. In defining property, Rousseau breaks society into two categories: the classes that own property and those that do not own property. Furthermore, since property is the engine of productivity, the latter should work for the former. Using this equation, government is the result of a contract made to maintain the privileges of the private property owners under the narrative of equality for all. Progress toward civilization made people slaves of society through dependence and competition over what we are and what we have. The purpose of politics, and thus of the state, is to restore balance—to reconcile rules and laws of collectivity. The social contract is about how we, as society, can live together, and for Rousseau we do so by submitting our individual will to the collective will.

Finally, in Rousseau's view, collectivity is different from an aggregation of individuals in that it has a common ground, or set of standards, that defines how the collective ought to be ruled by the sovereign. The sovereign emerges from this common ground that is itself the social contract. Submission to the general will implies duties from both parts: the sovereign is committed to each individual who helps the social contract emerge; and each individual is committed to the Other that represents the whole society through the sovereign. In the end, for Rousseau, the sovereign is both in charge of mediating the relation of duties and rights established by the general will and dependent on collective decisions and law.

Adam Smith, along with David Hume, is usually presented as utilitarian and therefore a critic of social contract theory. However, while Hume directly opposed the idea of the social contract on the basis of the fact that there is no actual point in history in which people agree to the social contract, Smith's critique has been more debated since there is no scholarly agreement on the position of utilitarianism or consequentialism.[6] Hume argues that the result of the relationship between the ruler and the ruled is the result of different types of cohesion and the duty of allegiance to one's government that derives from obedience rather than choice. For him, obedience was based on the potential to maximize individual utility, rather than to negotiate different interests, since choice was never free, and it always depended on access.[7] If not historical, then, what kind of agreement is the social contract? Willful consent is necessary to achieve a direct agreement, which, Hume argued, cannot be proved.[8] Thus, society deceives itself by creating a story of its obedience under the notion of a social contract that is, in fact, an agreement by inference that assumes *equal* capacity of choice. In reality, however, society is acting under terms of obedience to either natural or inherent authorities such as a god, a sovereign, or money.

On the other hand, Adam Smith offers an analysis of the relationship between the ruler and the ruled that is based on the different ways in which societies were organized. From this historical approach, he characterizes the relationships between government, people, and economy in different stages of society where structures, functioning, and living standards differ according to the various modes of production, property, and wealth.[9] Each mode of production required a different form of governing that defined the role of law at each stage of society. However, in every stage, government's main duty was to protect people either from violence or from oppression and injustice.[10] Smith's critique of the idea of a social contract is based on his understanding of political development as one product of the evolution of the relational condition of society in which economy is also one component of the human condition that helps define social and political structures. For Smith, the natural condition of this relationship was framed by the morality behind human actions that include both intentions and consequences.[11]

A broad range of scholarly work has pointed to Adam Smith's notion of a social contract based on the idea that agents in civil society attend to government in order to enhance a expected utility that will arise from following well-defined rules of morals. However, Smith based his views on justice and social contract theory on his understanding of the relational condition of the organization of society and more specifically in the duties of government. His criticism of Locke's version of social contract is based on its extreme focus on utility and the reduction of the state's role to the protection of rights. By linking the notion of morals to justice, Smith detaches the latter from its condition of natural right.[12] Using this distinction together with his understanding of human action as a moral intention leads Smith to not just moral consequences, therefore, but also to a role of state that securitized utility and expanded its authority to ensure some justice. For Smith this system of government is also a mechanism with which to negotiate the interests between market and society. Smith saw in the functioning of markets a natural tendency to seek equilibrium.[13] The government's role is to push that tendency toward the expected outcome (based on defined moral principles) and to define relational conditions of interdependence between intensions, actions, and consequences through institutional mechanisms.[14]

### Rawls and Gauthier on the Individual

By presenting a version of the social contract based on the rationality and morality of the individual, both John Rawls and David Gauthier effectively depoliticize the theory of the social contract. Rawls's theory of the social contract was based on a Kantian understanding of human reasoning and moral judgment where a moral and political point of view is achieved by impartiality and objectivity from the general point of view. Thus, these elements mediate the nature of justice and what it requires from individuals and from collective institutions. Following Kantian thinking, Rawls proposed that to choose principles for a more just society, the individual's social status, class, and so on would form a rational and impartial standpoint. Only through this rationality, argues Rawls, would it be possible to control the unfairness that emerges from knowledge of social difference. Such knowledge, he says, leads to prejudice, and such information inevitably leads to biased decision making. However, a rational person without such knowledge of specific circumstances will, by nature, choose the logical and rational position of balance without favoring anyone in particular. Thus, the "veil of ignorance" leads to a just decision since behind that veil everyone shares the same condition. In short, everyone becomes equal and, by adding no preconceived knowledge to rationality, everyone will reach the same logic conclusion regarding principles of justice. Rawls claims that the establishment of this notion of original position will settle "the question of justification . . . by working out a problem of deliberation."[15]

Rawls proposed two principles for his "theory of justice": everyone has as much liberty as he or she can grant to others; and social and economic advantages should be available to everyone, that is, access to the opportunity should be a universal event under conditions of unequal distribution (which can be just). These two principles are based on distribution. First is the distribution of liberty, and second is distributional access to social and economic goods. Further, these principles are achieved sequentially: the first one must be satisfied before moving to the second. It is this serial order of principles that, for Rawls, expresses rationality. For Rawls, justice itself is more fundamental as a principle than even the social contract. Indeed, it is this overriding sense of justice that defines the possibilities and limitation of the social construction of society. Justice, he claims expresses the very limitations of knowledge and the human condition. Celeste Friend points out that this is *the* most abstract version of social theory that nevertheless informs democracy and state policy.[16]

For Gauthier, the notion of social contract is based both on an understanding of social relationships as contractual ties that originated in human rationality and on a shared understanding of efficiency (in terms of maximizing utility). Rationality and shared understanding come, he says, from self-consciousness, which he understands as the "capacity of human beings to conceive themselves in relation to other humans, to human structures and institutions, and to the nonhuman or natural environment, and to act in the light of these conceived relationships."[17] This self-consciousness acts as individual morality and thus, there is no need for the external enforcement mechanism of the sovereign. Gauthier argues that rationality makes people stick to their agreements since these rational agreements are made for their advantage. Contrary to the concept of self-interest he argues that by serving the interest of the Other serves one's own interests, as well. Thus, by constraining our self to Others, the final outcome will be successful for all. The very action of constraining can vary from doing what the Other wants to acting in order to get a response from the Other. In both cases, the relation and interaction with the Other is what determines the possibility of maximizing self-interest. When morality is internalized, there is no need for a sovereign; the social contract for Gauthier is, therefore, based on the relational condition of the individual and the entire collective.

## THE SOCIAL CONTRACT AND CHANGE

Up to this point in this chapter, different versions of the social contract theory were constructed under the assumption of a universal individual. In each of these theories, difference is not relevant for the construction of a collective realm, For example, Rawls explicitly claimed the need to veil (or control) specific knowledge of difference in order to avoid prejudices. Contemporary critics of Rawls—mainly from feminist, critical theory, and race approaches—question the viability of this version of the social contract and the very definition of universality that is implied in such classic theories of social contract.

These critiques of universality bring the concept of *power* to the theory of social contract by asking key questions such as who defines the contract, how do power relations work in such a definition, and how do social and political institutions perpetuate relations of power (marriage, motherhood, etc.)? From this perspective, the social contract is based on our subjugation and inequality. The first question is *who* is the contractor? In modern theories, the contractor is assumed to be a universal and abstract individual disembodied from particular conditions of race, sex, class, culture, and so on. That abstract figure is portrayed as the representation of the majority, while in reality this theorized figure is an idealized image of those in places of power. For these more modernist approaches, only the ones in power can portray and define that universal image. The second question here is *what* informs the actions of the individual? For most modern theories, the rational human is concerned with maximizing his or her own individual interest. Thus, these theorists assume not only one universal contractor but also one universal and abstract interest.

These theories of social contract, based on a universal contractor with a universal interest, fail to represent the dynamic nature of human beings and society, not only in relation to differences in social place, geographies, and cultures, but also in terms of the very changing nature of the individuals. In short, contemporary critiques claim that social contract theories fail to represent the fullness of human psychology and motivations. These critiques also question the notion of freedom that is portrayed in different versions of the social contract, since humans enter into the social contract after coming from relations of dependency in the family and in society. Modern theories of social contract have defined a moral person. In so doing, they have also determined who counts as a full political being and who does not. This classification determines the worthiness of access, defines privilege, and creates the parameters of inclusion and exclusion that are manifested both formally and informally. Thus, inequalities based on difference (race, gender, class, disability, etc.) are not only a social construct but also a political one, fostered in part by the very notion of the social contract.

Since the contract is based on privileges that are the outcome of inequality, the social contract therefore allows for exploitation of both resources and people. It is not a hypothetical but an actual contract that society practices in everyday life that makes possible, justifying, and legitimizing, a *power* relationship within people and between people and their environment. These critiques point out how Western thinking has idealized the social contract as the way to live together in society without questioning the underlying implications of the very idea of a contract. Therefore, the social contract is a mechanism of inclusion and exclusion that represents the very structure of our current political and social systems.

## THE LINK TO ECONOMIC PERFORMANCE

The relationship between the rise of economic power and the social contract can be better understood by exploring the interaction between economics and politics and, further, the institutionalization of the economy as a power that influences the actions of the state or the sovereign. In an attempt to control the power of the sovereign, both modern and liberal paradigms propose a modern economy as the central mechanism of control. The rationality and predictability of the modern economy made it the proper instrument to achieve individual liberty that, consequently, led to collective well-being without the risk of the forceful despotism of the sovereign.

The shift to a more liberal worldview impacts not only the political dimension of modern society (or the urban) but also economic and social dimensions. This interwoven relationship between economics and politics is neither natural nor unintentional but it is a process in which both can debate, question, and re-create each other. The liberal ideology of individual materialism that claims the liberation of the individual to exercise entrepreneurial freedom is based on a strong belief in private property rights, a free market, and free trade—all essentially free from government interference. The role of the state within such a framework is then to create, preserve, and facilitate these freeing practices. The state assumes the responsibility to guarantee the quality and integrity of the market that will lead to the quality of life and integrity of individuals. In the case where the market does not exist, the role of the state is to create the market. The only legitimate option for the state is to protect individuals in the full enjoyment of their private rights.

When discussing the ideological foundations of such capitalist political economy we found Albert O. Hirschman especially useful. He looked specifically to the aspects that have ensured capitalism's success in contemporary world, particularly the ideological construction of self-interest. Originally presented as a way to escape the passion of rulers that led to absolutism, self-interest, argues Hirschman, became the spirit of capitalism. The initial conceptualization of interest included both economic and other human motivations, but the pursuit of *self*-interest implied the achievement of both profits and moral goals. The later isolation of the economic dimension and simplification of the concept of interest established a major transformation of the moral and ideological scene. This movement of ideas, Hirschman argues, is what has positioned economics at the center of the moral values of today's society. The idea of everybody contributing to the general welfare while pursuing their own self-interest implies unintentional achievement of collective welfare. The rationality and predictability of the modern economy made it the proper instrument to achieve individual liberty and, consequently, collective well-being.[18]

Two key moments that illustrate this institutionalization of economy as a central aspect in the renegotiation of the social contract in the United States are Alexander Hamilton's delivery of the *Report on Manufactures* to the U.S. Congress in 1791 and John Maynard Keynes's *The End of Laissez-Faire*, published in 1926.

## Alexander Hamilton

Secretary of the Treasury Alexander Hamilton's *Report on Manufactures*, delivered to the U.S. House of Representatives on December 5, 1791, is a classic document recommending economic policies aimed at stimulating the independence of the newly formed republic. Beyond its economistic policy recommendations, the report has often been cited as a prime example of how a social contract would work for the nation and the states. Hamilton's report was intended to position manufacturing as a key component in the productive scheme of the new nation. He argues that understanding the superiority of production over agriculture would produce better policies. Industry, he says, is portrayed as unproductive when, in reality, the opposite is true: the establishment and diffusion production would have a wide impact on labor and consequently on communities.[19] He identifies seven aspects in which the development of industry would have a more positive impact in society than agriculture division of labor, extension of the use of machinery, additional employment for underrepresented segments, the promotion of immigration, greater scope for diversity of talents and dispositions, more ample and various fields for enterprise, and the creation and securing of demand for the surplus.

Hamilton argues that a lack of vision in the new republic "confines their [the United States'] views to agriculture and refrains from manufacture" because of their perceived incapacity to compete equally with Europe.[20] He also claims that other nations were already attracting foreign capital for the purpose of developing industry, asking rhetorically why we should not also create advantageous policies in the new republic. However, in order for us to reach this stage of domestic industrial competitiveness, he proposes a range of state regulations and interventions that grant him a direct link to Rousseau's theory of social contract.[21] "To this day, the report is often heralded as the quintessential American statement against the *laissez-faire* doctrine of free trade and for activist government policies—including protectionist tariffs—to promote industrialization."[22] Most certainly, Hamilton's primary concerns were not with theorizing social contract but were more related to finding the mechanisms by which to ensure economic as well as political independence for the new republic. For this purpose, he elected to promote industry, instead of agriculture, as main source of the nation's wealth.

Hamilton argues that, left to itself, industry would naturally grow in the interest of the community, but he also points to the difficulties of starting new industries. He argues that in the initial stages of industry formation there is a role for government as a promoter and benefactor of these new manufacturing interests. Thus, public policy in the form of import duties, pecuniary bounties (subsidies), patents, and other mechanisms is meant to ensure the initial establishment of these new industries and their future, natural, prosperity, for the industry and humans. Hamilton's discourse, supporting the general policy of promoting industry as a means for economic growth and thereby improving the general welfare, goes a long way toward defining the role of the federal government in the economy of the new republic.[23] Using this foundational essay by Hamilton, we can see that, from this nascent stage in U.S. history, the intrinsic relationship between economy and politics is made evident. Here this relationship informs the idea of social contract in the United States by establishing not only the roles of parties and government as promoter or supporter of *individual* well-being but also the terms of the contract, once more legitimized in the name of the general welfare.

### John Maynard Keynes

A quarter into the twentieth century, at a moment in which there were more than a few cracks in Hamilton's relationship between politics and economics, a John Maynard Keynes essay proposed to consciously review the institutional and relational terms of the social contract. In *The End of Laissez-Faire*, published in 1926, he reviews various theories of the social contract before offering his own proposal. He starts by looking at the purpose of individualism as an alternative to the question of the authority of the monarch and of the church. This act, he claims, changes the ethics that until then had informed the very nature of the social contract through an acceptance of an individualistic, utilitarian approach that would later be extended to the whole of society.

As Keynes sees it, every transition to a new theory of social contract occurs in the name of equality and is justified by the idea of *collective* good. He criticizes Locke's version of equality because it is defined by property, which is itself a privilege. Keynes is critical of Rousseau's version of social contract equality because it is not a starting point but an outcome or a goal. And for Hume, the utilitarian argument "the greatest happiness of the greatest number" simply homogenizes the entire society. Keynes points out that, in all these different theories, there are important philosophical debates over the very concept of the social contract and the notion of private advantage to foster public good. This notion, for Keynes, is increasingly fundamental to the *politics* of the social contract. The idea of private advantage, he says, is institutionalized through the concept of laissez-faire, which is portrayed as the advantages gained when governments left trade alone: *to govern better, govern less.* The main Keynesian critique is that proponents of laissez-faire policy forgot that the political is intentional and that any preferred outcome requires specific actions in order to achieve it. Consequently, there is no such a thing as laissez-faire—it was and is a fantasy. Either you leverage or you hold, or you do both. These actions, Keynes argues, are *political* actions, they are intentional, and they are acts of *power.*

Keynes first reviews many of the assumptions of economic science. For him, economists choose a hypothesis closely related to the Darwinian notion of survival that is both simple and unreal: "It is a method of bringing the most successful profit-makers to the top by a ruthless struggle for survival, which selects the most efficient by the bankruptcy of the less efficient."[24] This hypothesis, he argues, considers not the process but only the final result, measured in terms of progress and efficiency, thereby creating a system that only allows those in the better positions to achieve the better outcomes. Keynes claims that the simplicity of the market hypothesis and the very logic of its theory make it universal and unquestionable, which therefore also makes it easy to forget the reality of the cities that are today characterized by informal, contested, and anchored economies.[25] The idea that independent growth unequivocally leads to collective development is based on the notion of addition that ignores the relational, unpredictable, and organic realities of society.

Keynes's argument also returns to the question of the role of the state in this relational and institutional context. He points out that defining what the state should care for and what it should leave for individual action has been "one of the finest problems in legislation." He argues that it is necessary to separate aspects that are part of the state agenda from aspects that are not in order to allow governments to accomplish their democratic principles. To achieve this division, Keynes proposes a series of strategies: first, that governments reorganize into smaller semiautonomous bodies whose foundational mission is to ensure public good. Second, that governments distinguish between social and individual (private) services in order to then focus on fulfilling the "functions which fall outside the sphere of the individual, to those decisions which are made by *no one* if the State does not make them."[26]

Keynes argues that many of the economic problems of his time resulted from the system allowing few to take advantage of possibilities that could affect a larger segment of the population. This he argues is a direct source of inequality. For Keynes, the solution to such inequality lies outside the individual realm, in institutions able to make use of data to engage in appropriate actions and control (i.e., governmental laws and policies). He suggests, for example, that governments establish policies to control the population size. His proposals were never intended to challenge capitalism. On the contrary, they were advanced to relationally re-create a political economy to correct its deficiencies. He wrote:

> These reflections have been directed towards possible improvements in the technique of modern capitalism by the agency of collective action. There is nothing in them which is seriously incompatible with what seems to me to be the essential characteristic of capitalism. . . . For my part I think that capitalism, wisely managed, can probably be made more efficient for attaining economic ends than any alternative system yet in sight, but that in itself it is in many ways extremely objectionable. Our problem is to work out a social organisation which shall be as efficient as possible without offending our notions of a satisfactory way of life.[27]

Keynes's strategy, therefore, can be seen as a way to save the market based on reproducing a set of laws for redistribution to make wider segments of society participate in the market. The answer, for Keynes, for the failure of the market is to insert *more* people—to reshape the role of state and ensure the effective participation of these people in the market. This new version of state is focused on the creation of laws to protect the ability of the market to function. Following this argument, it is then possible to challenge the notion of Keynes's contribution as anti-marketeer and rather propose an understanding of Keynes's pro-market approach since (he redefines the rules to maintain the hegemony of market, he reinforces state roles in protecting the market, and he seeks to create new markets and expands old ones.

In sum, Keynes's policy recommendations were intended to support the market after the Great Depression, and the only institution able to perform such a role was the state. For Keynes, the state would assume the responsibility for producing the physical as well as the organizational infrastructures that society needed to transform the individual capacity of the people of a society to participate into the market. Giving the state the role of ensuring the enlargement of individual purchasing power while regulating the relationship between the private and the people, opened a space for a vast majority of the population to consume more. Just as Keynes argued that utilitarian philosophy changed the nature of the social contract, this paper argues that the Keynesian strategy of using public expenditures to overcome market failure preceded consumerism in establishing a different version of the social contract. It defined a culture that privileged consumerism and materialism in the relationship between market and society.

## The Neoliberal Era

The modern increase in purchasing power has meant a major change in patterns of consumption and a subsequent increase in market growth due to a diversification of lifestyles. This, together with technological progress, has made possible a reduction in the prices of key goods and allowed more people access to more products and services that improve the material conditions of their lives. However, this exponential growth was caused by a disruption of forms of production brought on by new patterns of consumption—all of which could only occur for a fixed period of time. After this period of growth, a normal stabilization of the growth followed by stagnation historically has occurred causing a rearrangement of the interaction between state, markets and society. After the Keynesian stimulants, therefore, there has been a new round of the more conservative notions of expanded markets without rewarding failure. The shift from demand to supply has resulted in the institutional relations of political economy realigning so that the supply side is now considered to be the best policy way to ensure an increase in productivity. The reward to the supply side was mainly achieved at the expense of the benefits to individual demanders, more specifically of labor. The result, argues Piketty, is enhanced productivity because there is more labor available at less cost.[28]

The shift from Keynesianism to this new, more productive liberalism, or neoliberalism, may be the factor that, today, most influences another redefinition of the social contract. From the Keynesian approach that considered the irregularities and weaknesses of the market and proposed a strong and clear role for the government to the recycled notion of laissez-faire where the state again retracted to let the market grow essentially unimpeded, there has been a serious rearrangement of both the rights of individuals and the functions of the state. To illustrate this newest shift in the economic paradigm informing policy, political economist Thomas Palley has examined the differences between the different Keynesian schools in the United States and the United Kingdom. He argues that in terms of income distribution, U.S. neo-Keynesians align more closely to neoliberal principles, whereas U.K. post-Keynesians consider the significance of institutional factors, including bargaining power of different actors, to be important economic factors. Explicitly involving an understanding of power relationships moves the debate to the *political* sphere rather than the purely economic one. "For the 35 years after World War II (1945–1980), Keynesianism constituted the dominant paradigm for understanding the determination of economic activity. This was the era in which modern tools of monetary policy (control of interest rates) and fiscal policy (control of government spending and taxes) were developed. It was also a period in which union coverage rose to historical highs and 'New Deal' style institutions of social protection and regulation were expanded."[29]

This "new deal" did indeed change the structure of inequality, argues Piketty. But in general he finds that the richest 10 percent of population still owns 60 percent of the world's total wealth on average while the bottom 50 percent owns only around 2 percent. The redistribution of income and wealth that affected the middle 40 percent and the top 10 percent, allowing a patrimonial model of class to emerge, hardly impacted the bottom 50 percent. The question now is: to what extent has the emergence of this middle class changed the power structures and consequently the institutional arrangements in the world? In historical terms, the emergence of a middle class redefined not only the social landscape but also the political one. And the rise of the middle class implied the appearance of alternative lifestyles and alternative ideas of social values and democratic demands. The appearance of a middle class has transformed the reality of social mobility, allowing members of a segment of the population to improve their social rank based on skills and education rather than only on inherent wealth. This transformation in the social structure originated a change of perception about values for social development and the terms of the social contract.[30]

Returning for a moment to the mid-1970s, a broad set of questions about the sustainability of the Keynesian approach arose once again, leading to a new incantation about the virtues of the free market and deregulation, this time joined with a new narrative about the middle-class advantages of managerial and entrepreneurial approaches that favored efficiency and growth.[31] However, this approach was basically rooted in criticizing excessive state intervention and social protectionism. During the Keynesian era, the social contract was clearly related to employment and the security that accompanied it. The neoliberal turn directly condemned the Keynesian notion of full employment by expanding its implications for monetary and fiscal policies and consequently for general growth. The argument suggested that full employment could jeopardize opportunities for flexibility and entrepreneurial opportunity. In practice, this has meant that today labor policy has consistently promoted deregulation that has the potential to lead to higher inequalities, not only in terms of income but also in terms of quality of life. "For neoliberals, this is because the market is now paying people what they are worth; for post-Keynesians, it is because the balance of power in labor markets has tilted in favor of business."[32]

## THE CHANGING NATURE OF THE SOCIAL CONTRACT

Theories of social contract have been an important aspect of the debate about the state, its role, even its very nature and scope. To what extent should a state intervene in the construction and transformation of society? To what extent should it intervene in individual choice, either by granting access or adding choices? How far should it go in mediating the relationships between individuals and the collective? And, perhaps most important, how expansive should its involvement in economy be in order to ensure growth and development? These questions have been revisited in almost every re-creation of an active theory of the social contract. As this chapter demonstrates, how they are answered and acted upon can have serious practical effects on the formation and execution of state public policy. Recent debate about the social contract has frequently focused on labor, employment, and income policies that emphasize the economic dimensions of the relationship between society and the state. At present, the policy view is somewhat economistic—commodifying a political-economic relationship that now seems to be mediated by the market. Nonetheless, a number of other dimensions actually affect the relationship between the market and the state: health, education, environment, energy, infrastructure, and so on. All of these dimensions can be either individual or collective; some are both, such as health and education; and others are largely collective in nature, such as environment, energy, and public infrastructure. All of the dimensions we discuss have a social nature that inevitably attaches them to the public realm. The following sections propose aspects that could help link issues of health, environment, and energy to the current debate about a social contract.

### Health

Besides its individual dimension, health holds a collective dimension that affects social development. It also holds an educational dimension that is both individual and collective and is ultimately significant in the public policy arena. This implies a double consideration when discussing the relationship that defines the terms of the social contract and health. Traditionally considered a social service, health has been part of the responsibilities of the state; however, recent shifts in economic and political paradigms have led to a reinterpretation of the role of state that seems to be moving from that of provider to that of regulator. A key mediator between the relationship between social contract and health is education, specifically, educating everyone about the need for health to be available to all, not only in terms of access but also in terms of choice. This implies a necessary shift in the culture of health, a shift that will impact all public policies since food, environment, transportation, energy, and resources are all aspects that determine the options to be healthy. The right to health was the subject of article 25 of the Universal Declaration of Human Rights adopted by the United Nations in 1948.[33] The declaration represented a post–World War II international commitment to avoid the dramatic experiences of war. It was created as a roadmap for all nations to follow in order to guarantee the "equal and inalienable rights of all members of the human family."[34] Established during the same era, the World Health Organization (WHO) adopted its constitution the same year as the UN declaration. Nearly seventy years later, the principles put forth in these two documents seem even more relevant in the current context of globalization and economic (neoliberal) policies in which gaps and inequalities within and between countries have broadened.

The topic here involves more than the actual conditions of physical and mental health—it also involves the right to a condition of well-being that ensures that every person can fully participate in social activities such as work, schooling, and recreation. Thus, this notion of well-being cannot be determined solely through either discipline (in academia) or sector (in public policy) because every person adds daily activities of interconnectedness to education, environment, production, and so on. The right to health in article 25 also includes the right to an adequate standard of living. When the 1948 UN declaration was first adopted, economic, social, cultural, civil, and political rights were supposed to be equally important. However, in the aftermath of the Cold War, human rights and emphasis on certain rights following political worldviews led to key governmental dislocations. While Western world powers prioritized civil and political rights and described economic and social rights as aspirations, Eastern world powers maintained the opposite. This difference in approach preceded the implementation, in 1966, of two new agreements: the International Covenant on Economic, Social and Cultural Rights (ICESCR) and the International Covenant on Civil and Political Rights (ICCPR).[35]

The right to health in the ICESCR agreement referred to the right of all peoples to substantial elements of health such as medical care, access to health and well-being, and adequate infrastructure. The ICESCR right to health also contained freedoms and entitlements such as equality of access and provision (without any discrimination); the right to disease prevention, treatment and control; and the right to participate in health-related decision making at both national and community levels. However, the ICESCR agreement does not equate the right to health with the right to be healthy, since health is also influenced by factors that lay outside the control of the state.[36] Thus, the state can do only as much as possible to ensure the best possibilities according to its capacity and within its available resources.

The fact that the realization of the right to health is progressive depending on available resources imposes the regulatory need for continuous monitoring and evaluation. The progressive realization of standards to check the evaluative implementation of the right to health range among the following: health facilities, goods, and services on a nondiscriminatory basis; a minimum of essential food and safe drinking water; shelter, housing, and sanitation; and equitable distribution of health facilities, goods, and services.[37] The state's obligations to protect this right to health is, as we said, progressively realized, maintained, in reality, as these obligations are met by the capacity of the state. The question about the extent to which other actors in society have responsibilities with regard to the achievement of the right to health emerged in the 1980s with the advent of the HIV/AIDS crisis. This fact brought to the fore the interdependence and indivisibility of health with human rights. From this view, public health is just that—a public (collective) policy for everyone. In this context, health is presented as an integral dimension that includes not only social rights but also civil and political rights, such as freedom from stigma and discrimination and the rights to privacy, participation, and information.[38]

The 1990s marked another new era for the promotion and the protection of human rights. The World Conference on Human Rights in 1993 led the UN secretary general to establish a full UN reform program to face the challenges of the new millennium. In 2000, the UN Committee on Economic, Social and Cultural Rights expanded the interpretation of the right to health to include all the "underlying determinants of health": safe drinking water and adequate sanitation, safe food, adequate nutrition and housing, healthy working and environmental conditions, health-related education and information including information about sexual and reproductive health, and gender equality.[39] At the United Nations Millennium Development Summit that same year, 189 countries committed to engage in actions to fight against extreme poverty, hunger, and controllable diseases such as AIDS and malaria by 2015. These commitments constituted the eight Millennium Development

Goals (MDGs).[40] Although all the goals are interrelated and impact the right to health, four specifically target health problems: extreme hunger (MDG 1), child mortality (MDG 4), maternal mortality (MDG 5), and the spread of HIV/AIDS, malaria, and other diseases (MDG 6).

The ambition of the UN was to meet the Millennium Development Goals by 2015, and indeed progress has been made. What we see today is a dynamic panorama where the notion and definition of what actually entails the right to health has changed and expanded widely since the turn of the millennium. There now seems to be little debate about how, to what extent, the roles of the world's states and other social actors are changing. If we can say that more and more change is being progressively realized, what does it mean for the social contract?

### Environment

Until just a few decades ago, the world governments seemed to share an approach to the relationship between humans and nature that most of us would call global exploitation. Thus, a nation's development was founded on the maximum use of natural resources for economic growth. Following this view, under the industrialization model, the achievement of economic growth would automatically lead to improving the quality of life for everyone in a society. There is no doubt today that this approach severely damaged the environment, the results of which have caused many people to seek alternative approaches to development and concomitant aspirations for quality of life in different societies. Among many approaches to environmental degradation was the approach that development could be contextual. From this perspective, *human* development is diverse and situational and depends on *each* society—each supplying specific notions of quality of life and progress.[41] Two alternatives built from this view: a notion of development at human scale that proposed an individual idea of development based on different dimensions of personality, materiality, and the spiritual needs of individuals; and a notion of sustainable development that initially was employed to consider and conserve the foundational natural systems of human life but that quickly morphed into a more elaborate system of economic and social dimensions of human development.

Contemporary urban areas are facing complex challenges related to the rapidly changing processes of growth and urbanization. But, in the main, policy has not changed—government responses have traditionally emphasized economic approaches that aim to increase growth and promote global competitiveness, to the detriment of environmental and social concerns.

However, this approach has produced an uneven urban development characterized by increasing environmental damage and social inequalities. This has more recently led nations to consider policies that address more broadly the effects and causes of environmental degradation.

Recent world debates about the condition of the environment have led to a shift in global paradigms about development. Concerns about environmental degradation have been widely discussed. The first United Nations Conference on the Human Environment, held in Stockholm in 1972, recognized the need to look for common principles to guide actions addressing conservation and improvement of human environments. Environmental protection and upgrading were both presented as policy dimensions that directly affected people's well-being as well as their economic growth, but little change resulted. It took another two decades for the notion of human development and environmental degradation to find a global platform. In 1992 a second conference, "First Earth Summit," was held in Rio de Janeiro. This conference focused on the evaluation of previous commitments regarding the environment, current patterns of production and its impacts on environment, alternative energy and water sources, and transportation policies. At this summit, leaders of the attending governments committed to actions to conserve the world's forests, to enhance biodiversity, and to combat climate change and desertification. In sum, these topics became known as Agenda 21. The agenda was actually quite contextual and embraced topics such as global poverty, production, and consumption, as well as the sustainable management of natural resources.

Indeed, the pace of global action picked up after the Rio summit ended. In 1997, Rio +5 was held in New York City and in 2002 the Second Earth Summit (Rio +10) was held in Johannesburg. At that point, the world's national governments acknowledged both their limitations in achieving the 1992 goals and the need to redouble their efforts to protect the environment and implement policies toward a more sustainable development. A new definition of *development* also emerged at Rio +10, this time considering the need to balance economic growth with social development and environmental protection. These three dimensions were presented as the pillars of a much-expanded notion of sustainable development. Eight years later, aspects debated in these summits were included in the MDGs (see previous section), which openly declare the necessity of changing patterns of consumption and the use of natural resources—MDG 7 specifically aspires to environmental sustainability. Today it is important to ask different questions: In the last two decades of public debate and awareness about the need for environmental protection, what if anything, have we achieved? Has the world moved any closer to its goal of sustainable development that ensures increased quality of life for future generations? In short, has the world impacted public policy and therefore altered the terms of social contract in any way?

### Energy

Discussion about environmental impact can readily be refocused as a discussion about energy, which is an essential element of human life, and even more so for contemporary urban life. Often defined as the capacity to perform work, energy is what maintains life and thus any form of energy also impacts the environment. Clean energy, which has entered the debate as a key feature of sustainable development, not only has the ability to promote environmental protection but can also help with job creation and economic growth. Solar and other types of clean, alternative, energies are making great advances, not only in terms of their technological development but also in the ways they are positioned in the policy arena. Some claim that clean, energy-efficient, technologies are changing the patterns of energy consumption in specific areas. However, because the patterns of general consumption have not changed radically, the energy required for goods production and labor is still immense.

Advancing renewable sources of energy such as solar, wind, and hydroelectric has been part of the international energy debate since the Second Earth Summit in 2000. These forms of clean energy are low in carbon emissions and are mainly produced in place, thereby generating a relatively positive local impact. Although the transformation toward a low-carbon, in-place, economy seems technically possible, its costs in economic and political terms are still what define the scope of its implementation.[42] Of particular interest is how many countries today have access to alternative sources of energy and, in those nation-states, how many people have access to enough clean energy to cover even the basic activities of daily life, such as cooking, lighting, and commuting. The issue, then, is how nation-states create adequate public policies via the social contract that increase the access to clean, affordable, and safe sources of energy for a vast majority of people.

To address this issue, the German Advisory Council of Global Change (WBGU) recommends that world governments develop strategies for transformation toward a low-carbon economy by expanding their renewable energies. The WBGU argues that these forms of clean energy would have a positive impact on the mitigation of climate change. It further posits that alternative energies must be understood in a more complex and relational way and must be regulated globally to ensure sustainability. The WBGU also points out that limiting energy demand, primarily in industrialized countries, in terms of both production and consumption, is not especially difficult if all governments, markets, and societies apply themselves to the task.[43]

Put another way, reducing carbon emissions and lowering energy consumption impacts *all* aspects of life and, as noted earlier, implies a new type of social contract—one not just between state and society but also between society and market and between market and state. The productivity and consumption dimensions of the economic transformation we have discussed may be the weakest argumentative link. There is not just a need to build the case for the unproductive and unattractive features of climate damage, but the argument must also be built around the counter-attractiveness of renewable energies as competitive factors of capital accumulation. Therefore, today's social contract in regard to energy requires a global perspective that also recognizes the impacts of colonization and the consequent world segregation that colonization created and creates in the stages of development. Although developing countries today account for most of the energy demand,—this resulted from centuries of development (in developed countries), which in turn has resulted in domination by developed countries in production processes of restructuring and transformation. The WBGU argues that such dominance requires that developed countries now share in the global responsibility for long-term climate degradation.[44]

In terms of energy demand and energy transformation, it seems that if the current social contract—which one observer calls "the social contract of consumption" in which individual and collective well-being are determined by economic growth continues—then the current courses of increasing energy consumption and environmental degradation will collide.[45] In order to avoid such a collision, changes in energy consumption patterns will demand not only new technologies that use renewable sources of clean energy, but also a decisive new commitment from both state and market to make clean energy sources available and affordable in everyday life. Solving the issues of energy, environment, and—ultimately—health, will necessitate a new social contract, one built on both access to resources and means for individuals to make educated choices.

## BALANCING POLITICAL AND ECONOMIC POWERS

In sum, various arrangements of the social contract have been proposed at different times and under different relations between state, market, and society. From Hobbes to the present-day neoliberal critical perspectives, the social contract has been at the center of debates about social development.[46]

Ultimately, however, the social contract seems to be the structure—the scaffolding, if you will—of society as a collective enterprise. The notion of the collective has been central to the definition of government, and since the establishment of civil government (which has rules and directionalities), the collective framework has been defined by the notion of social contract. Each early theorist framed it a bit differently, but they all had a view on the collective. From Rousseau's starting point on the collective nature of the social contract, to Locke, with his notion of society as a collective of individuals, to Smith's view of best government as the one that provides the least amount of regulation, the social contract has been institutionalized through the relational condition of government as the mediating institution between the market and individuals. When the social contract has been debated, the relationship between freedom and rights of individuals has been the crucial point of difference. However, each of the early theorists suggests that these two attributes—freedoms and rights—can only be constructed *collectively* since they depend on some overarching structure that ensures their delivery and maintenance. This structure, or scaffolding, is provided by the state, which depends on interests and paradigms that have proposed different arrangements for the relationship among freedoms, rights, and equality.

A newer version of the arrangement was proposed from an understanding of a more organic relationship between the individual and social growth. This concept of natural equilibrium was promoted by Adam Smith. The equilibrating character of supply and demand could be attributed to the presence of Smith's "invisible hand" in the market place. This natural harmony would work the greatest good for the greatest number. Thus, the social contract, for Smith, was rearranged to ensure that the government should not intervene in the market because its intervention would destroy the organic relationship and the natural balance. Again moving rapidly into the twentieth century, rather than stimulate supply (à la Hamilton or Smith), John Maynard Keynes proposed to stimulate demand by radically transforming the notion of consumption and establishing it as a strategy to avoid overproduction. By altering patterns of consumption, Keynes embarked on a strategy to circumvent the failure of the market. The subsequent response from the supply side of the equation expanded production globally as well as consumption. By defining this new form of achieving the primary role of state of serving the market, Keynesians suggested that they had generated a new shift in the relationship between individuals and the market and individuals and states, therefore impacting the notion of the social contract.

In the main, these arrangements of the social contract have focused on individual liberty and on limiting the role of government to ensure the achievement of this liberty. The focus on individuals has an impact on the way we understand the social contract, introducing it as a key structural element of negotiation in the relationship between the market and society. Here the role of state vis-à-vis the market becomes critical. Today it is not possible to separate the discourse between the market and the state. Locke and Hume, as well as Smith's laissez-faire economics, essentially defend the idea that the market can ensure balance on its own and that the best role of the state is not to interfere, or to do so only to prevent market failure. After the dramatic economic recession and then the outright market depression, Keynes proposed to save the market from its own excesses by moving the institutional policy relationship from supply to demand. By ensuring against all-out market failure and socializing losses, the state was able to influence the purchasing power of the collective and increase collective dependency on consumerism. Later proposals by Friedrich Hayek and Milton Friedman returned to the notion that the market can be expanded without rewarding failure, therefore shifting the emphasis once again from the demand side to the supply side, in order to ensure an increase in productivity out of less labor at less cost per worker.

Understanding the social contract in these relational terms—between individual and collective, and between market and state—the question remains: what does the next version of the social contract look like? And related to that, under which parameters and in the service of whose interests will a new arrangement emerge? This task of balancing individual rights with collective needs requires a relational understanding that goes beyond the academic disciplines or institutional sectors. The interconnectedness of this balance mirrors the very nature of present society. Consequently, a shift in the contemporary notion of social contract will demand a recentering of the nexus of the dimensions of individual and collective that historically have been divided in theory and practice. Health, environment, and energy are not detached dimensions, so improvements in just one of them will not necessarily increase the quality of life for all, much less add to the contextual necessities of reducing poverty and increasing environmental education.

Social contract theories have most often focused on debates about the responsibilities of individuals in society. However, conditions today require that we move toward a more collective understanding of the contract. In this aftermath of the 2008 financial crash, environmental degradation and increased social inequality compel us to revisit the principles of the social contract in light of current economic and market principles for human development. What would the alternative theory be, then? Is it time for governments to step in and more fully assume their role as regulators in order to make the market more accountable for the market's effects on society and the environment? Is it time for civic society to engage in a new strategy of growth that overcomes the excessive emphasis on economic and individual dominance and advantage? Is it time for scholars to question the effectiveness of the credit and financial systems that have replaced the welfare state?[47] And, finally, what are the bases of the next version of the social contract?

## Notes

1. On Socrates, see Celeste Friend, "Social Contract Theory," *Internet Encyclopedia of Philosophy* (2004), accessed December 3, 2015, www.iep.utm.edu.

2. Although Hobbes referred to men's interests, we have updated the wording to be more inclusive.

3. Albert Hirschman, *The Passions and the Interests: Political Arguments for Capitalism Before Its Triumph* (Princeton, N.J.: Princeton University Press, 1977).

4. Hobbes quoted in ibid., 51.

5. John Locke, *Two Treatises of Government: An Essay Concerning the True Original, Extent, and End of Civil-Government*, parts 1–5 (1689), 116.

6. D. Collins, "The Fall of Business Ethics in Capitalist Society: Adam Smith Revisited," *Business Ethics Quarterly* 4 (1994): 519.

7. P. F. Brownsey, "Hume and the Social Contract," *Philosophical Quarterly* 28, no. 111 (April 1978): 132–48.

8. C. Chwaszcza, "Hume and the Social Contract: A Systematic Evaluation," *Rationality* 4 (2013).

9. G. Kennedy, "Adam Smith and the Role of the Metaphor of an Invisible Hand," *Economic Affairs* 31, no. 1 (2011): 53–57; J. Thrasher, "Adam Smith and the Social Contract," in *Adam Smith Review* 8 (2015).

10. D. Collins, "Adam Smith's Social Contract: The Proper Role of Individual Liberty and Government Intervention in 18th Century Society," Selected Papers from the 1988 Meeting of the Society for Business Ethics, *Business and Professional Ethics Journal* 7, nos. 3–4 (fall–winter 1988): 119–46.

11. Ibid.; Thrasher, "Adam Smith and the Social Contract."

12. E. Khalil, "Is Justice the Primary Feature of the State? Adam Smith's Critique of Social Contract Theory," *European Journal of Law and Economics* 6, no. 3 (1998): 215–30.

13. See also Ramesh Chandra, *Adam Smith and Competitive Equilibrium*, Strathclyde Discussion Papers in Economics No. 03-11, Department of Economics, University of Strathclyde, Glasgow, n.d.

14. A. Witztum, "Interdependence, the Invisible Hand, and Equilibrium in Adam Smith," *History of Political Economy* 42, no. 1 (2010): 155–92; J. B Wight, "The Treatment of Smith's Invisible Hand," *Journal of Economic Education* 38, no. 3 (2007): 341.

15. On Rawls's "veil of ignorance," see Friend, "Social Contract Theory." John A. Rawls, *Theory of Justice* (Cambridge, Mass.: Belknap Press of Harvard University Press, 1999 [1971]), 16.

16. Friend, "Social Contract Theory."

17. David Gauthier, "The Social Contract as Ideology," *Philosophy & Public Affairs* 6, no. 2 (winter 1977): 130–64.

18. Hirschman, *Passions and the Interests.*

19. Alexander Hamilton, *Report on the Subject of Manufactures* (1791), Speeches and Writings File, 1778–1804, box 24, reel 21, Alexander Hamilton Papers, Library of Congress, http://lcweb2.loc.gov.

20. Ibid.

21. Michael P. Federici, *The Political Philosophy of Alexander Hamilton* (Baltimore, Md.: Johns Hopkins University Press, 2012).

22. Douglas A. Irwin, "The Aftermath of Hamilton's 'Report on Manufactures,'" *Journal of Economic History* 64, no. 3 (September 2004): 800.

23. Ibid.

24. J. M. Keynes, *The End of Laissez-Faire* (London: L. & Virginia Woolf, 1926), accessed November 27, 2015, www.panarchy.org.

25. David C. Perry and Terry Mazany, eds., *Here for Good: Community Foundations as Foundations of Community* (Armonk, NY: M. E. Sharpe, 2014).

26. Keynes, *End of Laissez-Faire.*

27. Ibid.

28. Thomas Piketty, chapters 7 and 10 in *Capital in the Twenty-First Century*, translated by Arthur Goldhammer (Cambridge, Mass.: Harvard University Press, 2014).

29. Thomas I. Palley, "From Keynesianism to Neoliberalism: Shifting Paradigms in Economics Public Understandings of the Economy Also Matter," *Foreign Policy in Focus*, May 5, 2004, accessed November 27, 2015, http://fpif.org.

30. Piketty, chapters 7 and 10 in *Capital in the Twenty-First Century.*

31. David Harvey, "From Managerialism to Entrepreneurialism: The Transformation in Urban Governance in Late Capitalism," *Geografiska Annaler*, series B, *Human Geography* 71, no. 1, *The Roots of Geographical Change: 1973 to the Present* (1989): 3–17.

32. Palley, "From Keynesianism to Neoliberalism."

33. "(1) Everyone has the right to a standard of living adequate for the health and well-being of himself and of his family, including food, clothing, housing and medical care and necessary social services, and the right to security in the event of unemployment, sickness, disability, widowhood, old age or other lack of livelihood in circumstances beyond his control. (2) Motherhood and childhood are entitled to special care and assistance. All children, whether born in or out of wedlock, shall enjoy the same social protection." Article 25, "Universal Declaration of Human Rights," United Nations General Assembly resolution 217, December 10, 1948, accessed December, 3, 2015, www.un.org/en/.

34. Preamble in "Universal Declaration of Human Rights."

35. See Helena Nygren-Krug, WHO, "Health and Human Rights—A Historical Perspective," *UN Special* 673 (May 2008), accessed December 3, 2015, www.who.int/hhr.

36. International Covenant on Economic, Social and Cultural Rights (ratified December 16, 1966), Office of the United Nations High Commissioner for Human Rights (hereafter OHCHR), accessed December 3, 2015, www.ohchr.org/.

37. "The Right to the Highest Attainable Standard of Health: 11/08/2000. E/C.12/ 2000/4.(General comments)," CESCR, 2000, http://apps.who.int, accessed April 1, 2016.

38. "The Right to Health, Fact Sheet No. 31," OHCHR and World Health Organization, Geneva, June 2008, accessed December 3, 2015, www.ohchr.org.

39. "Right to the Highest Attainable Standard of Health."

40. UN, Millennium Development Goals and Beyond 2015, www.un.org/millennium goals.

41. G. Wilches-Chaux, ¿Y qué es eso, desarrollo sostenible? Cinco cuentos en la tienda y algunas herramientas en la trastienda para desarmarlos y volverlos a armar (Bogotá: Consejo Regional de Planificación, 1993).

42. "World in Transition: A Social Contract for Sustainability," German Advisory Council of Global Change (WBGU), Berlin, 2011, accessed December 3, 2015, www.wbgu.de/ en/home.

43. Ibid.

44. Ibid.

45. Bruce Jennings, "Beyond the Social Contract of Consumption," Minding Nature 2, no. 3 (2009), Center for Humans and Nature, accessed December 3, 2015, www.humans andnature.org.

46. David Harvey, A Brief History of Neoliberalism (Oxford: Oxford University Press, 2005); Jason Hackworth, The Neoliberal City Governance, Ideology, and Development in American Urbanism (Ithaca, N.Y.: Cornell University Press, 2006),

47. Robert Skidelsky, Keynes: The Return of the Master (New York: Public Affairs, 2010).

## Other References

Barkan, J. Corporate Sovereignty: Law and Government Under Capitalism. (Minneapolis: University of Minnesota Press, 2013).

Kennedy, G. "A Reply to Daniel Klein on Adam Smith and the Invisible Hand." Econ Journal Watch 6, no. 3 (2009): 374–88.

Kissinger, Deborah A. "Renegotiating the Social Contract: Hobbes to Rawls." Dissertation, University of Hawai'i, 2003.

Simpson, Matthew. "A Paradox of Sovereignty in Rousseau's Social Contract." Journal of Moral Philosophy 1 (2006): 45–56.

United Nations Department of Economic and Social Affairs. Renewable Energy. www.un.org/esa/desa/climatechange/renewableenergy.html.

United Nations Environment Programme. Declaration of the United Nations Conference on the Human Environment. 1972. www.unep.org/Documents.Multilingual/ Default.asp?documentid=97&articleid=1503.

Zimmerman, Aaron. "Hume's Reasons." Hume Studies 33, no. 2 (2007): 211–56.

PART TWO
# WHITE PAPERS

# Back to the Future?

## *The Curious Case of "Public" Services*

DAVID A. MCDONALD

QUEEN'S UNIVERSITY, CANADA

Modern networked services such as water, sanitation, and electricity have fluctuated back and forth between public and private ownership for more than 150 years. Most services in Europe and North America began as private entities, were municipalized and nationalized starting in the mid- to late 1800s, privatized again from the 1970s, and are now experiencing a (partial) shift back to public ownership and control.

This paper reviews the institutional scope and ideological character of these ownership swings, highlighting the diverse ways in which publicness has been expressed in service delivery and infrastructure. These past and present experiments demonstrate the dynamism and inventiveness of public service reform but also serve to illustrate how disjointed and contradictory conceptions of public services can be, and how easily notions of public and private can elide into one another. More recent efforts to claim public status for coproduction of services by non-state actors disrupts the historical state-private continuum but does little to resolve the inherent tensions behind what constitutes a public service.

The review is broken into four broad periods of service reform: early municipalizations (1850s–1930s), nationalizations (1930s–1970s), privatizations (from the 1980s); and re-municipalizations and renationalizations (after 2000). The intent of the paper is not to take a position on any particular form of public service provision but rather to demonstrate how complicated, ambiguous, and even misleading the moniker *public* can be. In doing so it underscores the tense yet symbiotic relationship between the state and private capital, with the latter relying to a large extent on the capacity of governments to facilitate capital accumulation via infrastructure development. Whether service delivery is public or private matters less than its instrumental outcomes, shaped in part by the competing interests of different factions of capital, as well as increasingly vocal and effective demands for input on decision making by citizens. Identifying a service simply as public does little to advance our understanding of what it is, who operates it, or in whose interests it has been established.

## EARLY MUNICIPALIZATIONS (1850s–1920s)

The rapid industrialization of European and North American cities in the 1800s witnessed a dramatic growth in large and small firms providing services for the productive and consumptive needs of a growing working and middle class. Water, gas, transportation, waste management, health care, and electricity services were among the networked amenities developed at that time, provided almost universally by private companies.[1]

Where economies of scale and capital intensity mattered (e.g., water and electricity), there tended to be larger (and increasingly oligopolistic) players, with some of the largest extant private utility companies owing their existence to this period (e.g., Suez, United Water, General Electric).[2] More localized services such as waste removal and health care were typically managed by small, sometimes informal, private providers, although consolidations quickly became the norm.[3]

This laissez-faire approach to service development began to change in the mid- to late 1800s with a push to *municipalize* facilities—that is, having a local state authority take ownership and control of services. This trend spread throughout Europe and North America and carried into the 1940s.[4] The overarching rationale for municipalization was that service provision by multiple providers was illogical and wasteful, particularly with so-called natural monopolies such as water, gas, and electricity, for which it made little economic or regulatory sense to have duplicated personnel and infrastructure.

Outbreaks of cholera and other public health concerns added to the pressure. The British Parliament passed a series of public health measures as early as 1848 mandating local authorities to take action. Sanitary reformers had exposed the gross inadequacies of a noninterventionist approach that had allowed nine companies in London to partition the water supply among themselves in what became a "nine-headed monopoly."[5] It proved impossible to regulate them all, and none of these firms was clearly tasked with supplying water for other critical municipal purposes, such as firefighting.[6]

Similar concerns were raised with capital-intensive services such as transportation, gas, and electricity, but the municipalization movement came to encompass an extraordinary range of public services. England alone had public enterprises numbering in the hundreds, including slaughterhouses, cemeteries, crematoria, libraries, refuse and sewage disposal services, a printing plant, a sterilized milk depot, and a wool conditioning house. Leisure activities were also commonly provided for and included aquariums, boys' clubs, parks, public baths, racecourses, and theaters.[7]

This state-owned enthusiasm nevertheless hid competing and often inconsistent ideological motivations for municipal takeover. On the left, some advocates of municipal socialism advanced a strong anticapitalist sentiment— even in the United States, where, at the peak of the Socialist Party in the early 1900s, "about 1200 party members held public office in 340 cities, including seventy-nine mayors in cities such as Milwaukee, Buffalo, Minneapolis, Reading, and Schenectady."[8] This brand of municipalization ridiculed the Robber Barons of the day, with explicit commitments to fairness and universal access based on "widespread anti-monopoly sentiment" that "flowed easily into calls for public production and distribution of basic goods and service."[9] As Dreier notes of this time: "Progressive reformers fought alongside radical socialists to champion child labor laws, women's suffrage, and the establishment of public hospitals and clinics while leashing the power of landlords, banks, railroads, and utility companies."[10]

But just how socialist this movement was is disputed. Many critics saw these initiatives as too compromised—practically and ideologically—to create real social and economic change, with no less a detractor than Vladimir Lenin declaring the municipalization trend to be incapable of bringing about larger socialist transformation. These far-left critics disdained the gradualist municipal politics of the Fabians, rejecting the parliamentary road to socialism that they said gas-and-water enterprises represented. "The bourgeois intelligentsia", continued Lenin, "elevate municipal socialism to a special 'trend' precisely because it dreams of social peace, of class conciliation, and seeks to divert public attention away from the fundamental questions of the economic system as a whole, and of the state *structure* as a whole, to minor questions of local self-government."[11]

To the right were pro-market liberals who argued for municipalization on efficiency grounds, in part to combat the municipal socialist movement. Economist John Stuart Mill, for example, took up the cause of water reform in Britain, criticizing the wastefulness of balkanized private supply. In 1851, he thought it obvious that great savings in labor "would be obtained if London were supplied by a single gas or water company instead of the existing plurality. . . . Were there only one establishment, it could make lower charges, consistently with obtaining the rate of profit now realised." It was an error, he argued, to believe that competition among utility companies actually kept prices down. Collusion was the inevitable result, not cheaper prices. Nor was water the only service that would be most efficiently provided by a single supplier. Mill also pointed out the benefits of centralization in "the making of roads and bridges, the paving, lighting, and cleansing of streets."[12]

Similar arguments were made in the United States, where the commitment to municipal services was more a response to the corruption and ineffectiveness of private companies than any ideological strategy. There were, in fact, Republicans who ran and served as reform mayors.[13] These pro-market municipalizers were exemplified by the goo-goos (short for "good government") of Chicago in the early 1900s, whose "chief interest was to introduce honesty and business-like efficiency into city government. Believers in individualism, the Protestant work ethic, and private enterprise, they strove for a municipal authority that, once cleansed of corruption, would be smaller in size and function and would guarantee lower taxes and enforcement of public order and private morality" (much like advocates of 'new public management' today, as discussed below).[14]

As such, it can be argued that the outcome (if not always the intent) of this initial wave of municipalization was to reinvigorate capital accumulation, not to challenge it—a form of state capitalism that was to be a precursor to a more highly theorized, scaled-up and explicitly antisocialist Keynesian project from the 1930s. Recognizing the inefficiencies and health dangers of fragmented private supply systems, policy makers and certain factions of capital saw municipalization as the most immediate and effective way to prevent market decay and enhance market opportunities. As MacKillop notes in the case of early water infrastructure in Los Angeles, "public investments furthered private interests on a grand scale," as land developers pushed for public service extension to open new frontiers of accumulation. Capitalists allowed municipal socialism to develop and thrive, but only insofar as it suited their needs: "Nobody wanted this [municipalization] venture to be too ideological or harmful to private enterprise. . . . The idea was to make the municipal water service [in Los Angeles] work efficiently, to ensure the city's 'greatness,' and without harm to the city's financial situation. As long as this didn't prevent the oligarchy from making money, they didn't object."[15]

The colonial experience with municipalization, it should be noted, was very different. British administrative councils in southern Africa, for example, had no pretense of serving the public as a whole. The municipalization of the water supply in Johannesburg in 1905 was prompted as much by the water requirements of the mines as by those of white city residents. And Johannesburg chose to run its water service at a profit rather than lowering the price, which would have encouraged consumption by poorer inhabitants.[16]

Moreover, public health crises were often used by colonial authorities to justify the mass removals of non-Europeans from central city locations rather than expand public services. In what has been dubbed the sanitation syndrome, white municipal administrations throughout Africa blamed epidemics on urban Africans to rationalize the destruction of their housing and the creation of segregated cities, even though the rhetoric was one of municipalization for improved *public* services.[17]

## SCALING UP IN THE KEYNESIAN ERA (1930s–1970s)

From the 1930s and escalating rapidly in the 1940s, we see a winding down of the municipalization movement (particularly for nonessential services such as restaurants and theaters) and a scaling up of larger, networked state services to the national and regional levels.[18] Much of the latter occurred in sectors where new technologies and modes of governance made large, networked services possible, such as with electricity and health care. Water provision, by contrast, stayed largely at the municipal level due to transportation costs, although policy and regulation were partly scaled up.

This nationalization trend was part of a larger paradigm shift in Western market economies at the time, with expanded public services seen as an essential part of a nationally coordinated stimulus package for production and consumption to recover from economic downswings (Keynesianism and the welfare state), and for building national competitive advantage (Fordism).[19] Combined with the growing authority and capacity of central states—driven in part by the demands of big business for centralized bargaining—the rationale of service efficiency and strategic planning that drove municipalization was now being employed in the nationalization agenda to "ensure that the commanding heights of the economy remained in public hands and was subject to government directions."[20]

The shift from municipal to national state ownership was particularly dramatic in Britain. In the early 1940s, roughly 30 percent of local government income was generated by locally-owned public services. Three decades later this had been whittled down to less than 2 percent.[21] In the electricity sector, 65 percent of British local authorities supplied their own power, but these were nationalized at the stroke of a pen when more than six hundred power producers were rolled into a single national authority by the Electricity

Act of 1947.[22] By the 1960s, national-level public expenditures accounted for approximately 60 percent of gross national product, and a fifth of all goods and services were under national public ownership.[23]

Meanwhile, ostensibly nonessential services such as markets and municipal restaurants disappeared altogether, often vilified as creating unfair competition and stifling entrepreneurship, leaving the field open to private enterprise. In effect, the emergence of *national* welfare states took the wind out of *municipal* public service sails, advancing capital accumulation on an increasingly national and even global scale while squashing the potential for more radical redistributive initiatives locally.

By the 1970s, this nationalization project was hegemonic, prompting Milton Friedman's derisive quotation at the height of welfarism's influence that "We are all Keynesians now."[24] The scale and pace of nationalization differed from place to place—as did the character of state welfare spending—but the trend toward national public ownership of key services was widespread throughout Western market economies.[25]

The trend was pervasive in newly independent postcolonial states, as well. Those not allied to the Soviet bloc invariably introduced some form of welfare service provision via new state-owned enterprises or nationalized private entities left over from the colonial era, with the aim of accelerating development objectives that the market on its own would not be able to satisfy (with the dual aim of creating a domestic capitalist class).[26]

The range and quality of these public services varied dramatically, depending on state capacity, colonial legacies, and ideological makeups. Some regions (notably Latin America) initiated the state enterprise project earlier and more enthusiastically, while others (notably sub-Saharan Africa) suffered from massive skills and infrastructure deficits that made large-scale service delivery projects difficult. In virtually all cases, however, public services catered largely to an urban elite, lacking the accumulation incentives to extend state resources to an underemployed and under-consuming mass. As a result, state-owned services, whether local or national, seldom resulted in universal or equitable provision, although the official justification for state ownership was to make services available to all.

## BACK TO PRIVATE (FROM THE 1980s)

By the 1970s, a simmering backlash against state ownership broke out of its academic confines and into the public realm with the election (and imposition) of neoliberal governments around the world, starting with the United

Kingdom (Margaret Thatcher) and Chile (Augusto Pinochet). This neoliberal transition is well documented and need not detain us here, but it is worth reviewing the fundamental arguments behind the rationale for returning (in part) to private-sector provision of essential services more than a century after the private ownership model had come under attack.

Essentially, neoliberals argued that state ownership of key services had outlived their usefulness to become a drag on, rather than a stimulant for, economic growth. Lacking financial incentives to perform efficiently or respond to user demands, state employees were deemed to have become sclerotic and unaccountable, creating distant, unimaginative services that were out of touch with local populations and unable to respond to the needs of a dynamic private sector in a rapidly changing and highly competitive global market economy.[27]

Privatization, by contrast, offered the benefits of better responsiveness to market demands and improved accountability by dint of transparent contracts that revealed the true costs and benefits of service delivery. The result was to be a more efficient use of resources, lower service costs for end users, more choices for consumers, improved awareness of different service needs, and more rapid economic growth for all by facilitating the expansion of infrastructure required for a modern mass consumption society. Privatization was also seen as pro-poor, insofar as it ensured cost recovery for sustainable provision and expansion of services, and creative delivery by entrepreneurs that could target the affordability levels of different income groups. This was not a promise of immediate parity but one of incremental progress that would ignite a virtuous cycle of growth and create (local) private sector jobs without overtaxing an economy's growth engines.[28]

This is classical liberal economic theory at heart—with the assumption that human beings are inherently self-interested utility maximizers that respond best to financial (dis)incentives in a market economy. But this renewed push for privatization is also *neo*-liberal in the sense that it advances a more robust role for the state than did the laissez-faire governments of the nineteenth century—not necessarily in size, but in terms of government's capacity to develop policy, monitor change, and regulate service delivery performance by the private sector. And although initial waves of neoliberal privatizations saw some wholesale divestitures of public services—such as water and sanitation facilities in the United Kingdom and Chile—for the most part so-called privatization has been composed of public-private partnerships (PPPs) where the state retains some ownership or management role, or both, in contracts with private companies.[29]

It is also neoliberal in the sense that this new vision of service provision focuses on states at the local level once again, with an explicit agenda of decentralization and denationalization, ostensibly to democratize policy making by bringing decision making to the lowest, closest level to those that it serves. Good governance—as this framework has come to be known—was intended to resolve the problems of market failure that John Stuart Mill had identified in the nineteenth century. With the right regulations, it is argued, virtually *any* public good can be provided by the private sector, as described by Joseph Stiglitz: "If regulated and monitored well, and perhaps if subsidized to some extent, public goods and services can be produced by markets while still retaining their public consumption properties. While public support will have to be greater for goods or services destined to serve the poor, even poverty reduction programs can be implemented through public-private partnering and incentive schemes that allow private actors to take the extra step of adjusting their behavior to generate social (public) benefits as well as adequate private returns."[30] As such, recent forms of privatization are only a partial return to the past. They convey not an abandonment of the state but rather a mix of entrepreneurial private capital with the command and control effects of state involvement, lending credence to the argument that the last three decades of reform have been as much a process of neo-Keynesianism as of neoliberalism.[31]

## BACK TO PUBLIC? (AFTER 2000)

Since the turn of the new millennium we are witnessing what appears to be yet another reversal, with renewed interest and growth in state-owned enterprises around the world.[32] Does this shift represent the demise of privatization? Are we seeing a return to older forms of state ownership? Are there new dynamics at play?

The answer to these questions is "yes and no." In some respects, contemporary experiences with re-municipalization and renationalization mimic the institutional and ideological rationales for state provision of the past, but they also introduce new elements to an otherwise simplistic public-private binary, with the introduction of non-state actors such as community groups in the coproduction of services, the use of legislative mechanisms to prohibit privatization, more democratic forms of socialism, and a host of other pragmatic forms of public service provision.

In the following I identify four distinct (though not unrelated) motivations for a return to state provision of essential services, including several important subcategories. Although every case is different, there are broad undercurrents that we can use to identify and heuristically categorize this recent back-to-public trend. I start with the most overtly anti-privatization of these, moving through categories that may or may not be ideologically opposed to private sector participation, finishing with a discussion of corporatization, a form of state ownership that can be as commercial as outright privatization and which is sometimes little more than preparation for future private-sector involvement.

### Overt Opposition to Privatization

Given the intense debates around privatization over the past thirty years, it comes as little surprise that one of the rationales for returning to (or retaining) state ownership has been explicit opposition to private-sector participation in essential services. Some of this opposition has been overtly anticapitalist in its orientation, as with the renationalization and restructuring of multiple service sectors in Bolivia and Venezuela, from energy to communications. In these cases, privatization is argued to be an extension of an inherently unequal market system and therefore fundamentally incapable of providing equitable and sustainable service delivery. But rather than adopting Soviet-style centralization, these governments have developed various forms of twenty-first-century socialism, intended to be more democratic and participatory, working with grassroots demands for social control of essential services.[33]

In other cases, anti-privatization sentiment has played itself out in more social democratic fashion. In Uruguay, for example, the government has recently nationalized or strengthened state ownership of a wide range of services, although it remains firmly committed to a broader market economy.[34] An illustration of this was a referendum held during the 2004 national elections to amend the country's constitution to make private provision of water and sanitation services illegal, stipulating that these services must be provided directly by the state.[35] This was the first such constitutional amendment in the world, winning the support of 62 percent of voters, at the same time as it saw the election of a leftist coalition party (Frente Amplio) for the first time in Uruguay's 170-year history.

Several other countries have subsequently used legalistic strategies to attempt to oppose privatization. In Italy, anti-privatization activists won a reverse victory of sorts in 2011, defeating a law introduced by Silvio Berlusconi's government that sought to privatize all public services of economic significance, including water. In this case, a national referendum saw the defeat of the proposed legislation by a margin of 96 percent, although it did not outlaw privatization per se.[36] A similar law was recently revoked in Indonesia, which had previously allowed the private sector to monopolize water resources.[37] Similar initiatives have been taking place at the municipal level. In 2011, residents of Berlin (Germany) voted by a margin of more than 98 percent to pass a draft bill to force the municipal administration to disclose secret agreements on the partial privatization of the city's water services.[38]

Importantly, none of these legal initiatives has managed to ban privatization. Even Uruguay still has private water companies operating in the country under its new constitution.[39] Nor are these examples anti-capitalist per se. What they have done is to put a damper on privatization initiatives and strengthened the possibility of state-driven service reform, including greater democratization and citizen participation in decision making.

### Pragmatic Publics

Much less political has been the trend to make services public again on financial grounds, mostly at the municipal level. In these cases, municipal bureaucrats recognize that in-house service provision is less expensive and less complicated than outsourcing or privatizing. The transaction costs of private-sector participation in essential services can be considerable in terms of managing contracts and overseeing quality control, forcing many municipalities to ask if privatization makes economic sense.[40]

The city of Paris remunicipalized its water services for these reasons in 2010, calculating that it could reduce financial and monitoring costs by providing water in-house. The fact that Veolia and Suez lost the contract—two French multinational water companies that had been operating the city's water on contract for the previous twenty-five years and had been active in water provision in Paris since 1860—made this remunicipalization a particularly symbolic event, but the driving force was not ideological. There was an immediate €35 million cost saving to the municipality the first year, an 8 percent reduction in water tariffs for end users, and an integration of hitherto fragmented portions of the water system (making it easier to manage).[41] And although the initial impetus for the remunicipalization had come from a Socialist Party mayor almost a decade earlier, the process to bring it to fruition was a largely bureaucratic one, with most Parisians unaware of the take over until it had (seamlessly) transitioned to a new municipal entity on January 1, 2010.

Similarly bureaucratic decision-making processes characterize much of the remunicipalization trend in the United States, where state delivery accounts for almost half of all local government services on average, and where insourcing (as re-municipalization is known in the United States) has been on the increase for the past decade or more.[42] Here, as well, privatization reversals are a reflection of a pragmatic desire to employ cost-saving reforms that bureaucrats deem to work, as opposed to any particular commitment to notions of publicness.

## Impromptu Publics

In other cases, the return of services to the state has been unplanned—even unintentional—lacking any clear practical or ideological vision. One reason for this has been sudden cancellations of long-term private contracts or unilateral departures of private companies, or both. In Buenos Aires, for example, French multinational Suez had been granted a thirty-year concession to run the city's water and sanitation services in 1993, but years of poor performance, combined with the collapse of the Argentine economy and its currency in 2001, led to an abrupt termination of the contract by the national government and a protracted period of painful stop-start negotiations among federal officials, the municipality, foreign governments, international tribunals, workers' unions, and Suez.[43] The end result was the formation of a new state-owned water company in 2006. This organization has managed to introduce more affordable water rates, expand services and infrastructure, and make itself more transparent and participatory than Suez. However, none of these reforms had been thought through in advance, and significant performance concerns remain. These problems are due in part to some of the institutional legacies of the privatization era but also stem from the ad hoc and unprepared ways in which the renationalization process took place, despite a government that was formally committed to a state-led macroeconomic agenda.[44]

Similar dynamics have played themselves out in Cochabamba, Bolivia, where the U.S. water company Bechtel was chased out of the city by massive anti-privatization protests in 2001. The local and national governments at that time were in favor of privatization and therefore unprepared for what to do next, but even after the election of the Movement for Socialism (MAS) party in 2005, reforms have been haphazard. Almost fifteen years on, Cochabamba is still struggling to rebuild an effective post-privatization water provider, hobbled in part by the institutional legacies of the past, as well as radically different visions of what a public water provider should look like—a democratically healthy, but institutionally exhausting and tension-laden dynamic.[45]

Unexpected returns to state ownership have also occurred when there have been a lack of (credible) bidders on private contracts. In these cases, the state has indicated its desire for private-sector participation in services and issued a call for proposals, but private firms have not bid because the contract conditions are either deemed too strict (often in countries in the Global North) or because the investment is seen as too financially risky (often in low-income countries in the Global South). The City of Hamilton, Canada, for example, signed a ten-year concession for water services with a private company in 1994. When the contract came up for renewal, the municipality tightened up its demands for contract performance (notably environmental standards), but no private bidders were willing to meet the new expectations. The city was then forced to bring water services back in-house, despite a strong pro-privatization sentiment among managers and city council members. Despite this, the re-municipalization process has resulted in an improvement in the quality and transparency of services, and there appears to be little impetus to reprivatize water at this time, although the city continues to contract out other services and has increasingly commercialized its water and sanitation operations since returning them to public hands.[46]

In Dar es Salaam, a very different process resulted in a similar remunicipal-ization outcome. Under intense pressure from the World Bank, the government of Tanzania agreed to a ten-year lease contract with a British-German consortium to operate the city's water and sanitation services. The process of finding private companies willing to operate in a city with such decrepit water infrastructure and high rates of poverty was itself problematic (and secretive—even the Tanzanian Parliament was unaware of the contract nego-tiations until they were finalized—suggesting problems from the start). The contract was canceled a mere twenty-one months later. The police arrested the company's executives and expelled them from the country for repeated violations of the contract. Plans to find new private bidders were quickly dropped, with the World Bank instead pushing for a re-municipalization of the city's water services on the grounds that suitable bidders would not be found. Dar es Salaam Water and Sewerage Corporation is now owned and operated by the Tanzanian state, but with conditions imposed by the World Bank that the public company must be run on private-sector principles with a focus on cost recovery and financially based performance evaluations.[47]

### Corporatization

This last example offers a segue into what has arguably been the most com-mon form of public-service delivery over the past thirty years: corporatization. Sometimes described as agencies or parastatals, corporatized entities are fully owned and operated by the state but have a degree of autonomy from government. They typically have a separate legal status from other public-service providers and a corporate structure similar to publicly traded private-sector companies, such as a board of directors.

Corporatized entities currently "make up the bulk of the public sphere in many Western European countries" and are increasingly popular in the South.[48] China has arguably been the most active on this front, converting thousands of its state-owned enterprises into arm's-length agencies.[49] Water and electricity utilities are common examples, although the practice extends to a much wider range of services, including airports, child care, universities, forests, hospitals, and transportation.[50]

The institutional objective of corporatization is to create arm's-length enterprises with independent managers responsible solely for the operation of their own immediate organization, where all costs and revenues are accounted for as though they were stand-alone companies. This ring fencing is intended to create greater financial transparency, reduce political interference, and strengthen managerial accountability within relatively autonomous service entities. It can also serve to enhance the borrowing status and credit ratings of agencies less encumbered by complex intra-governmental finances.

More controversially, corporatization has been used to create market-friendly public-sector cultures and ideologies. Since the late 1970s, corporatized public utilities have been run increasingly on market-oriented operating principles such as financialized performance indicators, cost-reflexive pricing, and competitive outsourcing—part of a larger neoliberal trend toward so-called new public management. Proponents of this model celebrate market-based management techniques as an effective way to depoliticize public services and improve efficiency.[51] It is here that we hear the echoes of the goo-goos of Chicago a century ago, whose chief interest in making municipal services public was to bring a businesslike efficiency into city government.

In some cases, corporatization goes a step further, with the express intent of outright privatization once the profit potential of a ring-fenced entity has been realized and market-based accounting structures and management cultures are in place. In other cases, governments may corporatize as an interim strategy during recessionary times, waiting for a better opportunity to privatize.[52]

Corporatization may be public in name, therefore, but not necessarily in character, raising questions about the substance and nature of state ownership under this public model and whether it differs from more direct forms of private-sector participation. Some critics see corporatization as the proverbial wolf in sheep's clothing, offering a facade of public ownership while propagating market ideology and advancing corporate accumulation—achieving the same goals as privatization without the political and financial risks associated with it.

For their part, corporatized managers can adopt zealous market-oriented styles, languages, and techniques, often pushing through policies and actions (e.g., widespread water cutoffs to low-income families) that private companies would not implement themselves for fear of public backlash. As a result, corporatization has seen a growing emphasis on cost-reflexive pricing and expenditure reductions via outsourcing as well as other discreet forms of cost cutting. Consumers are increasingly seen (and come to see themselves) as customers instead of citizens, with services seen as commodities to be bought and sold like any other product on the market, dissociated from broader public goods and concealing the complex social and labor arrangements behind their exchange price.[53]

Another concern is the institutional myopia created by corporatization. Under welfarist forms of public administration, different services were typically connected via horizontally organized departments. With the advent of neoliberal corporatization, they have been legally and physically separated from one another and told not to waste resources on other government agencies, contributing to a blinkered approach to service planning and delivery. As a result, corporatized entities can operate in splendid isolation from one another, even if they share the same equipment and serve the same population, often becoming fiefdoms with protective barriers erected in the name of autonomy.[54] Competition within and across service units becomes valorized, typically requiring deregulation of monopolistic state control and allowing multiple service providers to compete for subcontracts based on price.

Not all corporatizations have been carried out with this commercial imperative in mind, however. The seemingly singular administrative structure of corporatization belies more diverse material and philosophical undercurrents, from proto-privatization to distributive welfarism, some of which have been remarkably progressive.[55] In Costa Rica, for example, ICE (the electricity utility) has been one of the most efficiently run companies in all of Latin America, public or private, while still retaining a commitment to universality and equity. Their record is based in part on a long history of commitment to public service, embedded in the social democratic characteristics of Costa Rica's *modelo solidario* (solidarity model). ICE has occupied an important place historically in the configuration of national social identity and has been shaped by specific political, social, and economic conditions. Costa Rican citizens are aware of the state's contributions to national development and have proudly resisted previous attempts to privatize public enterprises. ICE is seen as a driver of social and economic progress and has been at the center of some of the most important social mobilizations of the past.[56]

Tunisia's state-owned electricity provider, Société Tunisienne de l'Électricité et du Gaz (STEG), offers another, though very different, illustration of relatively progressive corporatization. Founded in 1962, STEG has been enormously successful at extending affordable and reliable electricity and gas services throughout the country, without relying on harsh cost recovery policies. With more than 99 percent coverage in both rural and urban areas, STEG has created the highest level of access to electricity in all of Africa. Much of this was accomplished under an autocratic regime, however, and although there are ongoing efforts to democratize STEG in the post–Arab Spring era this will not be an easy task given its long history of cloistered management. Nevertheless, STEG leaders continue to resist pressures to privatize, and the company remains in public hands.[57]

## LESSONS LEARNED

What lessons can we draw from 150 years of public-private oscillation? One message is that we should not put too much stock in the value of the words themselves. So-called public services can operate much the same way as private companies, celebrating their public status when the situation demands and exploiting their private potential when it does not. The large number of transnational public enterprises that defend their public standing at home while operating on a for-profit basis overseas is illustrative of this dual personality.[58]

One such example is Manitoba Hydro (Canada), which is fighting off a privatization attempt from within its own province while having been awarded a contract to privatize the electricity transmission network of Nigeria.[59] State-owned Rand Water and Eskom in South Africa have done the same, as have Vattenfall (Sweden), EPM (Colombia), and Huaneng Power (China), to name but a few public agencies that appear, for all intents and purposes, as private, for-profit corporations outside their borders.[60]

There is also the growing use of public-sector union pension funds to invest in the privatization of public services. The Ontario Teachers' Pension Plan, for example, owns a controlling share of the water and sanitation services of Chile (originally privatized under Pinochet), even though the teachers' union whose members pay into the fund holds strong anti-privatization policy positions in Canada. Publicly owned sovereign wealth funds are also investing in privatized infrastructure.[61] Such is the curious case of so-called public services today.

Part of the problem here is a poverty of language. The word *public* is decidedly unqualified for defining an extremely diverse and complex set of realities on the ground—as is its apparent binary, *private*. In reality, the public is composed of an intricate web of private individuals and organizations, all with an influence on collective outcomes, and vice versa. To speak of a "public service" tells us little about any single agency's ontological status or its intended outcomes.

Perhaps it is best to think of *publics*—in the plural—recognizing both the complex ways in which different forms of public services come together and the very dissimilar outcomes they can produce. In this regard, we may need multiple forms of measuring success, recognizing a core set of universal principles that all public services could aim for (e.g., equity, accountability, sustainability) while at the same time acknowledging that no two places and sectors will value performance in exactly the same ways.[62]

The emergence of non-state, nonprofit actors in modern networked services disrupts the public-private dualism further still. Whether by choice or by default, community groups, NGOs, unions, and others are playing an increasingly large role in the delivery of essential services, either on their own or in partnership with governments. The practice ranges from organized informal waste pickers in India to faith-based hospitals in rural Uganda to community-owned water aqueducts in Colombia, covering everything from participatory budgeting to worker co-ops.[63]

One must be careful not to fetishize community participation, of course. Non-state actors may have much to contribute to the development of more democratic forms of service delivery, but they are not necessarily "the most reliable sources of social innovation," as some advocates argue, and are unlikely to have the financial or organizational capacity to resolve the massive service backlogs that exist, particularly in countries in the Global South.[64] There is also the danger that community participation will be co-opted by neoliberal policy makers in an effort to download the physical and financial costs of service provision onto (poor) communities.[65]

Ironically, the more robust these debates about alternatives to privatization become, the harder it is to develop a coherent pro-public movement. Anti-privatization sentiment has been remarkably consistent over the past thirty years, but these agreements hide deep differences of opinion as to what should take its place. Nor should we expect widespread agreement on alternative visions of what it means to be public any time soon, given the chasms in differences of opinion.[66]

In this respect, we can take a cue from Ferguson, who asks what happens if politics is not just about "expressing indignation or denouncing the powerful. What if it is, instead, about getting what you want? Then we progressives must ask: what do we want? This is a quite different question (and a far more difficult question) than: what are we against?"[67] History tells us much about the nature of public–private swings in the past, but we have much more to learn about where new forms of public services might take us in the future.

## Notes

1. W. M. Emmons, "Private and Public Responses to Market Failure in the US Electric Power Industry, 1882–1942," *Journal of Economic History* 51, no. 2 (1991): 452–54; M. V. Melosi, *The Sanitary City: Environmental Services in Urban America from Colonial Times to the Present* (Baltimore, Md.: Johns Hopkins University Press, 2000); M. V. Melosi, *Garbage in the Cities: Refuse Reform and the Environment* (Pittsburgh: University of Pittsburgh Press, 2005); S. B. Warner, *The Private City: Philadelphia in Three Periods of Its Growth* (Philadelphia: University of Pennsylvania Press, 1987).

2. M. Granovetter and P. McGuire, "The Making of an Industry: Electricity in the United States," *Sociological Review* 46, no. S1 (1998): 147–73; D. Lorrain, "La firme locale–globale: Lyonnaise des Eaux (1980–2004)," *Sociologie du Travail* 47, no. 3 (2005): 340–61.

3. Melosi, *Sanitary City*; G. Rosen, *A History of Public Health* (Baltimore, Md.: Johns Hopkins University Press, 1993).

4. D. E. Booth, "Municipal Socialism and City Government Reform: The Milwaukee Experience, 1910–1940," *Journal of Urban History* 12, no. 51 (1985): 225–35; W. C. Crofts, *Municipal Socialism* (London: Liberty and Property Defence League, 1895); J. R. Kellett, "Municipal Socialism, Enterprise and Trading in the Victorian City," *Urban History* 5 (1978): 36–45.

5. R. A. Lewis, *Edwin Chadwick and the Public Health Movement* (London: Longmans Green, 1952), 57.

6. The irrationality of the London model is captured mockingly in the Hollywood film *Gangs of New York*, where rival firefighting groups fist-fight over who has the right to put out a fire while the building in question burns.

7. E. Leopold and D. A. McDonald, "Municipal Socialism Then and Now: Some Lessons for the Global South," *Third World Quarterly* 33, no. 10 (2012): 1837–53.

8. P. Dreier, "Radicals in City Hall: An American Tradition," *Dissent*, December 2013, accessed May 3, 2015, at www.dissentmagazine.org; see also I. Graicer, "Red Vienna and Municipal Socialism in Tel Aviv 1925–1928," *Journal of Historical Geography* 15,

no. 4 (1989): 385–402; M. Fechner, "Municipal Socialism in Germany since the War," *Labour Magazine* 8 (1929): 364–67.

9. G. Radford, "From Municipal Socialism to Public Authorities: Institutional Factors in the Shaping of American Public Enterprise." *Journal of American History* 90, no. 3 (2003): 863–90.

10. Dreier, "Radicals in City Hall." See also D. P. Nord, "The Paradox of Municipal Reform in the Late Nineteenth Century," *Wisconsin Magazine of History* 66 (1982): 128–42; Radford, "From Municipal Socialism to Public Authorities."

11. V. I. Lenin, "The Agrarian Programme of Social-Democracy in the First Russian Revolution, 1905–1907" (1907), accessed December 12, 2009, at www.marxists.org.

12. J. S. Mill, "The Regulation of the London Water Supply" (1851), in J. M. Robson, ed., *The Collected Works of John Stuart Mill*, vol. 5, *Essays on Economics and Society Part 2* (Toronto: University of Toronto Press, 1967), 88, accessed July 8, 2009, at http://oll.libertyfund.org.

13. Radford, "From Municipal Socialism to Public Authorities."

14. R. A. Morten, "Public Transportation and the Failure of Municipal Socialism in Chicago, 1905–07," *Illinois History Teacher* 9, no. 1 (2002): 28–36; see also J. L. Merriner, *Grafters and Goo Goos: Corruption and Reform in Chicago, 1833–2003* (Carbondale: Southern Illinois University Press, 2004).

15. F. MacKillop, "The Los Angeles 'Oligarchy' and the Governance of Water and Power Networks: The Making of a Municipal Utility Based on Market Principles (1902–1930)," *Flux* 60–61 (2005): 23–34.

16. J. P. R. Maud, *City Government: The Johannesburg Experiment* (Oxford, U.K.: Clarendon Press, 1938), 130.

17. M. W. Swanson, "The Sanitation Syndrome: Bubonic Plague and Urban Native Policy in the Cape Colony, 1900–1909," *Journal of African History* 18, no. 3 (1977): 388–89.

18. R. Millward, "The 1940s Nationalizations in Britain: Means to an End or the Means of Production?," *Economic History Review* 50, no. 2 (1997): 209–34; D. L. Morton, "Reviewing the History of Electric Power and Electrification," *Endeavour* 26, no. 2 (2002): 60–63.

19. David Harvey, *The Limits to Capital* (London: Verso, 1982); B. Jessop, "Liberalism, Neo-Liberalism and Urban Governance: A State Theoretical Perspective," *Antipode* 34, no. 3 (2002): 452–72.

20. Y. Aharoni, "Charting the Iceberg: Visible and Invisible Aspects of Government," in *Evaluating the Welfare State: Social and Political Perspectives*, ed. S. E. Spiro and E. Yuchtman-Yaar, 161–75 (Oxford, U.K.: Elsevier, 2013).

21. J. Sheldrake, *Municipal Socialism* (Avebury, U.K.: Aldershot, 1989), 18.

22. J. Cheshire, "UK Electricity under Public Ownership," in *The British Electricity Experiment: Privatization: The Record, the Issues, the Lessons*, ed. J. Surrey, ch. 2(New York: Routledge, 2013), Kindle edition.

23. Aharoni, "Charting the Iceberg," 162.

24. Milton Friedman quoted in "The Economy: We Are All Keynesians Now," *Time*, December 31, 1965; see also Milton Friedman, letter to the editor, *Time*, February 4, 1966.

25. G. Esping-Andersen, *The Three Worlds of Welfare Capitalism* (Cambridge, U.K.: Polity Press, 1990).

26. K. Sanyal, *Rethinking Capitalist Development: Primitive Accumulation, Governmentality and Post-Colonial Capitalism* (New York: Routledge, 2014); J. Sender and S. Smith, *The Development of Capitalism in Africa* (New York: Routledge, 2013).

27. T. J. Biersteker, "Reducing the Role of the State in the Economy: A Conceptual Exploration of IMF and World Bank Prescriptions," *International Studies Quarterly*, 1990, 477–92; I. W. Lieberman, "Privatization: The Theme of the 1990s," *Columbia Journal of World Business* 28, no. 1 (1993): 8–17; J. Williamson, "What Washington Means by Policy Reform," *Latin American Adjustment: How Much Has Happened* 7 (1990): 7–20.

28. World Bank, "World Development Report 2002: Building Institutions for Markets" (Washington, D.C.: World Bank, 2002); World Bank, "World Development Report 2004: Making Services Work for Poor People" (Washington, D.C.: World Bank, 2003).

29. K. Bakker, "The Ambiguity of Community: Debating Alternatives to Private-Sector Provision of Urban Water Supply," *Water Alternatives* 1, no. 2 (2008): 236–52.

30. J. E. Stiglitz, prologue, in *The New Public Finance: Responding to Global Challenges*, ed. I. Kaul and P. Conceição, xii–xv (Oxford: Oxford University Press, 2006).

31. A. Saad-Filho and D. Johnston, eds., *Neoliberalism: A Critical Reader* (London: Pluto Press, 2005).

32. D. Chavez and S. Torres, eds., *Reorienting Development: State-Owned Enterprises in Latin America and the World* (Amsterdam: Transnational Institute, 2014); S. Clò, C. Del Bo, M. Ferraris, and M. Florio, "Mapping Public Enterprises in the New Millennium: A Participatory Research Database," paper presented at the Public Enterprises in the 21st Century conference, CIRIEC International, Berlin, Germany, February 14–15, 2013; M. Florio, *Network Industries and Social Welfare: The Experiment that Reshuffled European Utilities* (Oxford: Oxford University Press, 2013).

33. A. Kennemore and G. Weeks, "Twenty-First Century Socialism? The Elusive Search for a Post-Neoliberal Development Model in Bolivia and Ecuador," *Bulletin of Latin American Research* 30, no. 3 (2011): 267–81; D. L. Raby, *Democracy and Revolution: Latin America and Socialism Today* (London: Pluto, 2006).

34. D. Chavez and S. Torres, eds., *Reorienting Development*.

35. P. Terhorst, M. Olivera, and A. Dwinell, "Social Movements, Left Governments, and the Limits of Water Sector Reform in Latin America's Left Turn," *Latin American Perspectives* 40, no. 4 (2013): 55–69.

36. J. Dugard and K. Drage, "Shields and Swords: Legal Tools for Public Water," Occasional Paper No. 17, Municipal Services Project, Cape Town, 2012.

37. F. S. Sundaryani, "Court Bans Monopoly on Water Resources," *Jakarta Post*, February 20, 2015, accessed March 20, 2015, at www.thejakartapost.com.

38. R. Beveridge, F. Hüesker, and M. Naumann, "From Post-Politics to a Politics of Possibility? Unravelling the Privatization of the Berlin Water Company," *Geoforum* 51 (2014): 66–74.

39. S. Spronk, C. Crespo, and M. Olivera, "Modernization and the Boundaries of Public Water in Uruguay," in *Rethinking Corporatization and Public Services in the Global South*, D. A. McDonald, ed., 107–35 (London: Zed Books, 2014).

40. A. Hefetz and M. E. Warner, "Contracting or Public Delivery? The Importance of Service, Market and Management Characteristics," *Journal of Public Administration Research and Theory* 22, no. 2 (2012): 289–317.

41. M. Pigeon, "From Fiasco to DAWASCO: Remunicipalising Water Systems in Dar es Salaam, Tanzania," in *Remunicipalisation: Putting Water Back into Public Hands*, ed. M. Pigeon, D. A. McDonald, O. Hoedeman, and S. Kishimoto, 40–57 (Amsterdam: TNI, 2012).

42. A. Hefetz and M. E. Warner, "Privatization and Its Reverse: Explaining the Dynamics of the Government Contracting Process," *Journal of Public Administration, Research and Theory* 14, no. 2 (2004): 171–90; G. C. Homsy and M. E. Warner, "Intermunicipal Cooperation: The Growing Reform," in *The Municipal Yearbook 2014* (Washington, D.C.: International City County Management Association, 2014).

43. A. J. Loftus and D. A. McDonald, "Of Liquid Dreams: A Political Ecology of Water Privatization in Buenos Aires," *Environment and Urbanization* 13, no. 2 (2001): 179–99.

44. D. Azpiazu and J. E. Castro, "Aguas Públicas: Buenos Aires in Muddled Waters," in Pigeon et al., *Remunicipalisation*, 58–73.

45. N. Laurie, "Gender Water Networks: Femininity and Masculinity in Water Politics in Bolivia." *International Journal of Urban and Regional Research* 35, no. 1 (2011): 172–188; A. J. Marston, "Autonomy in a Post-Neoliberal Era: Community Water Governance in Cochabamba, Bolivia," *Geoforum*, 2013, doi.org/10.1016/j.geoforum.2013.08.013; M. Olivera, "Water Beyond the State," *NACLA Report on the Americas* 47, no. 3 (2014): 64.

46. M. Pigeon, "Who Takes the Risks? Water Remunicipalisation in Hamilton, Canada," in Pigeon et al., *Remunicipalisation*, 74–89.

47. B. Dill and B. Crow, "The Colonial Roots of Inequality: Access to Water in Urban East Africa," *Water International* 39, no. 2 (2014): 187–200; Pigeon, "From Fiasco to DAWASCO."

48. W. J. M. Kickert, "Public Management of Hybrid Organizations: Governance of Quasi-Autonomous Executive Agencies," *International Public Management Journal* 4, no. 2 (2001): 135–50; see also J. Alvarez, "Privatization of State-Owned Agricultural Enterprises in Post-Transition Cuba," *Problems of Post-Communism* 53, no. 6 (2006): 30–45; C. Benzing, "Cuba—Is the 'Special Period' Really Over?," *International Advances in Economic Research* 11, no. 1 (2005): 69–82; I. Bremmer, "State Capitalism

Comes of Age: The End of the Free Market?," *Foreign Affairs*, 2009, 40–55; D. Chavez and B. Goldfrank, *The Left in the City* (London: Latin American Bureau, 2004).

49. V. A. Aivazian, Y. Ge, and J. Qui, "Can Corporatization Improve the Performance of State-Owned Enterprises Even without Privatization?," *Journal of Corporate Finance* 11, no. 5 (2005): 791–808; J. Ocko and L. Campo, "Focus on the Corporatization Process in China," *Duke Journal of Comparative and International Law* 5 (1994): 145; M. Ramesh and E. Araral, "Reasserting the Role of the State in Public Services," in *Reasserting the Public in Public Services: New Public Management Reforms*, ed. M. Ramesh, E. Araral Jr., and X. Wu, 1–16 (New York: Routledge, 2010).

50. Aivazian, Ge, and Qui, "Can Corporatization Improve the Performance of State-Owned Enterprises Even without Privatization?"; N. Bilodeau, C. Laurin, and A. Vining, "Choice of Organizational Form Makes a Real Difference: The Impact of Corporatization on Government Agencies in Canada," *Journal of Public Administration Research and Theory* 17, no. 1 (2007): 119–47; H. D. Meyer, "The New Managerialism in Education Management: Corporatization or Organizational Learning?," *Journal of Educational Administration* 40, no. 6 (2002): 534–51; D. P. Moynihan, "Ambiguity in Policy Lessons: The Agencification Experience," *Public Administration* 84, no. 4 (2006): 1029–50; H. W. Nelson and W. Nikolakis, "How Does Corporatization Improve the Performance of Government Agencies? Lessons from the Restructuring of State-Owned Forest Agencies in Australia," *International Public Management Journal* 15, no. 3 (2012): 364–91; T. H. Oum, N. Adler, and C. Yu, "Privatization, Corporatization, Ownership Forms and Their Effects on the Performance of the World's Major Airports," *Journal of Air Transport Management* 12, no. 3 (2006): 109–21; A. S. Preker and A. Harding, *Innovations in Health Service Delivery: The Corporatization of Public Hospitals* (Washington, D.C.: World Bank, 2003); J. Sumsion, "The Corporatization of Australian Childcare: Towards an Ethical Audit and Research Agenda," *Journal of Early Childhood Research* 4 (2006): 99–120; A. Zatti, "New Organizational Models in European Local Public Transport: From Myth to Reality," *Annals of Public and Cooperative Economics* 83 (2012): 533–59.

51. C. Hood, "A Public Management for All Seasons?," *Public Administration* 69, no. 1 (1991): 3–19; Organisation for Economic Co-operation and Development, *OECD Guidelines on Corporate Governance of State-Owned Enterprises* (Paris: OECD Publishing, 2005); D. Osborne, and T. Gaebler, *Reinventing Government: How the Entrepreneurial Spirit is Transforming the Public Sector* (Reading, Mass.: Addison-Wesley, 1992); Preker and Harding, *Innovations in Health Service Delivery*; M. M. Shirley, "Bureaucrats in Business: The Roles of Privatization Versus Corporatization in State-Owned Enterprise Reform," *World Development* 27, no. 1 (1999): 115–36.

52. Aivazian, Ge, and Qui, "Can Corporatization Improve the Performance of State-Owned Enterprises Even without Privatization?," 791; Florio, *Network Industries and Social Welfare*.

53. J. Clarke, J. Newman, N. Smith, E. Vidler, and L. Westmarland, *Creating Citizen-Consumers: Changing Publics and Changing Public Services* (Thousand Oaks, Calif.: Sage Publications, 2007).

54. D. Bollier, *Silent Theft: The Private Plunder of Our Common Wealth* (London: Routledge, 2002); M. J. Whincop, ed., *From Bureaucracy to Business Enterprise: Legal and Policy Issues in the Transformation of Government Services* (Aldershot, U.K.: Ashgate, 2003).

55. See, for example, the cases in McDonald, *Rethinking Corporatization and Public Services in the Global South*.

56. D. Chavez, "An Exceptional Electricity Company in an Atypical Social Democracy: Costa Rica's ICE," in McDonald, *Rethinking Corporatization and Public Services in the Global South*, 31–61.

57. A. Bennasr and E. Verdeil, "An 'Arab Spring' for Corporatization? Tunisia's National Electricity Company (STEG)," in McDonald, *Rethinking Corporatization and Public Services in the Global South*, 88–106.

58. J. Clifton, F. Comin, and D. Diaz-Fuentes, eds., *Transforming Public Service Enterprises in Europe and North America: Networks, Integration and Transnationalisation* (New York: Palgrave, 2007).

59. S. Price, "Public Utilities Exporting Privatization," *Dominion*, April 2014, accessed January 21, 2015, at http://dominion.mediacoop.ca.

60. K. Furlong, "Water and the Entrepreneurial City: The Territorial Expansion of Public Utility Companies from Colombia and the Netherlands," *Geoforum* 58 (2015): 195–207; L. Gentle, "Escom to Eskom: From Racial Keynesian Capitalism to Neo-Liberalism (1910–1994)," in *Electric Capitalism: Recolonizing Africa on the Power Grid*, ed. D. A. McDonald, 50–72 (London: Earthscan, 2009); J. Monstadt, "Urban Governance and the Transition of Energy Systems: Institutional Change and Shifting Energy and Climate Policies in Berlin," *International Journal of Urban and Regional Research* 31, no. 2 (2007): 326–43; C. van Rooyen and D. Hall, "Public Is as Private Does: The Confused Case of Rand Water in South Africa," MSP Occasional Paper No. 15, Municipal Services Project, Cape Town, 2007.

61. R. D. Lipschutz and S. T. Romano, "The Cupboard Is Full: Public Finance for Public Services in the Global South," Occasional Paper No. 16, Municipal Services Project, Cape Town, 2012.

62. See D. A. McDonald and G. Ruiters, eds., *Alternatives to Privatization: Public Options for Essential Services in the Global South* (New York: Routledge, 2012).

63. G. Baiocchi and E. Ganuza, "Participatory Budgeting as If Emancipation Mattered," *Politics and Society* 42, no. 1 (2014): 29–50; M. Bélanger Dumontier, S. Spronk, and A. Murray, "The Work of the Ants: Labour and Community Reinventing Public Water in Colombia," Occasional Paper No, 28, Municipal Services Project, Cape Town, 2014; Spronk, Crespo, and Olivera, "Modernization and the Boundaries of Public Water in Uruguay"; P. Chikarmane, "Integrating Waste Pickers into Municipal Solid Waste Management in Pune, India," in *Pune, India: Women in Informal*

*Employment Globalizing and Organizing* (New Delhi: WIEGO, 2012); D. Hall and E. Lobina, "Water as a Public Service," Report for PSI, Public Services International Research Unit, London, December 15, 2006, accessed September 10, 2012, at http://gala.gre.ac.uk; Y. M. Dambisya, M. Manenzhe, and A. B. Kibwika-Muyinda, "Faith-Based Health Services as an Alternative to Privatization? A Ugandan Case Study," Occasional Paper No, 25 Municipal Services Project, Cape Town, 2014.

64. J. McCarthy, "Commons as Counterhegemonic Projects," *Capitalism Nature Socialism* 16, no. 1 (2005): 9–24.

65. B. Jessop, *The Capitalist State: Marxist Theories and Methods* (Oxford, U.K.: Martin Robertson, 1982).

66. D. A. McDonald, "Building a Global Pro-Public Movement," in *Making Public in a Privatized World: The Struggle for Essential Services*, ed. D. A. McDonald (London: Zed Books, 2016).

67. J. Ferguson, "The Uses of Neoliberalism," *Antipode* 41, no. S1 (2009): 166–84.

# The History of U.S. Municipal Service Delivery

## *Pragmatism Trumps Ideology*

DISCUSSANT: DENNIS R. JUDD
UNIVERSITY OF ILLINOIS AT CHICAGO

In his chapter, "Back to the Future? The Curious Case of 'Public' Services," David McDonald provides a cogent analysis of the long history of "public" services provided by municipal governments. He places the word "public" in quotation marks because, as he notes, the definition of that important term has been slippery, changeable, and increasingly murky over time. In his account, until at least the mid-nineteenth century most municipal services in Europe and North America were provided through private entities, but over time governments stepped in as major providers. In the twentieth century, a push for nationalizing services that began in the 1930s moved the balance to the so-called public side of the ledger; beginning in the 1980s, a movement toward privatization shifted the scale in the other direction. In the current period, coproduction and corporatization, which range widely from full privatization in profit-making entities to progressive organizations committed to goals of equity, the public-private boundary often becomes very opaque.

Despite the difficulties of marking off the ambiguous boundaries between the public and private realms, debates over how to provide services have often been cast in ideological terms that assumed that a stark distinction could be made. Two periods, in particular, bear this out; but, I argue, a U.S. culture of pragmatism has always tended to shove things toward a middle ground. The movement to municipalize services during the Progressive Era serves an excellent example.

Without doubt, the Progressive Era campaign to assert public control over privately run services was informed by a national revolt against the corruption of the public realm by the robber barons of that era. Self-identified socialists won the mayor's office in several major cities, but *socialist* is an overly ambitious term for many of the reforms they implemented. The campaigns to reign in the power of utility and traction companies, for example, generally focused on regulating rates and levels of services, and municipal ownership was pursued only when more limited measures proved to be inadequate. Ohio mayors Tom L. Johnson of Cleveland (1901–09), Samuel "Golden Rule" Jones of Toledo (1897–1903), and Brand Whitlock of Toledo (1906–13) all won election by fighting against high streetcar and utility rates, and for fair taxation and better social services. Their campaigns became models for like-minded reformers elsewhere. Reform-oriented mayors in Jersey City, Philadelphia, and Cincinnati also renegotiated streetcar and utility franchises, measures that fell short of municipal ownership.[1]

The career of Hazen S. Pingree, who served as Detroit's mayor from 1890 to 1898 and later as governor of Michigan, shows how mixed the reforms, and the institutional fixes, were even when reform was very aggressively sought. Pingree was picked as the Republican candidate for mayor in 1889, mostly because the exclusive Michigan Club who not persuade any of its other members to run. The business leaders who controlled Republican politics trusted him, as a member of the club, to advocate the usual program of low taxes and a minimal array of municipal services, but when Pingree won the election he was shocked at what he found: one of the worst street systems in the nation, a ferry service that charged usurious rates, and a streetcar system that refused to convert to electric power. The new mayor threatened to revoke the ferry company's charter if it did not cut rates, and he removed it from some of the choice waterfront property it occupied.

Pingree's fight with the Detroit City Railway Company turned especially bitter when he backed an employee strike against the company and refused management's request to call in the state militia. He declared that privately owned public services were "the chief source of corruption in city governments."[2] The company demanded that the city negotiate a more favorable franchise, but Pingree countered with a lawsuit meant to terminate the existing company in favor of municipal ownership. Ultimately, both he and the company accepted a regulatory regime that gave the mayor most of what he wanted. By 1895, however, Detroit began operating a municipal electric plant to supply power for its streetlights, which ended a five-year running battle between Pingree and the private lighting company. He also initiated a protracted battle to force the Detroit Gas Company to lower its natural gas rates; ultimately, the company gave in. To fight Bell Telephone Company, Pingree chartered a publicly owned phone company; within a few years Bell bought it out, but lowered its rates and improved its services.

Thus, reform took many paths even within a single city, as it also did across the nation. In the industrial cities, Progressive and even Socialist ideals provided a rough guide to reform, but as Amy Bridges's pioneering research shows, urban reform in southwestern cities was almost solely motivated by a desire of local elites to establish institutions capable of supporting rapid economic and population growth. As a consequence, the independent public agencies that emerged to dredge harbors, build transportation systems, or provide services were tightly controlled by local elites.[3]

The arrangements for providing services also remained highly variable in a later period of reform that seemed driven by ideological concerns. In 1992 Osborne and Gaebler published *Reinventing Government*, which seemed to capture perfectly the zeitgeist of the antigovernment campaigns of the Reagan presidency.[4] Osborne and Gaebler proposed that privatizing a whole array of city services could make services more efficient and effective by putting them on a business footing. Within a few years, many cities instituted competitive bidding procedures that put the private sector into competition with city agencies. Cities across the nation adopted contracting out as a best practice for cutting costs and improving service performance.

However, we must avoid jumping to conclusions about how much this movement represented a particular ideological agenda. Democratic mayors, for example, were eager to adopt any sensible practices that might reduce the cost of municipal services. Chicago's six-term mayor, Richard M. Daley, made this clear in a *New York Times* op-ed published just weeks after his 1991 reelection: "we've introduced privatization in city government, and the innovation hasn't been nearly as distasteful as many predicted. In this union town, there were plenty of skeptics. But privatization has worked—with bumps. . . . City government should stick to basic services it provides very well and buy others. It matters little to the tax-paying public, which expects good service,

who renders it." In a *Business Forum* op-ed, Daley declared that "Privatization
. . . recasts government as more of an overseer than a provider—the guard-
ian of the public well-being instead of the source. Fulfilling this new, more
sophisticated role requires new skills of government employees. They have
to sit down with private-sector professionals and set performance standards."
Following Daley's example, Republican mayor Richard Riordan of Los Angeles and Democratic mayor Ed Rendell of Philadelphia also aggressively
pursued privatization.[5]

The motive of pure pragmatism can be observed, once again, in the present
era. Beginning in the 1980s, a generation of visionary mayors pioneered in
the creation of institutions capable of financing and administering projects
considered important for promoting the economic viability of inner cities.
Thus, sports authorities were created for the purpose of building sports stadiums, mall authorities were incorporated to build and administer mall and
entertainment complexes, and development corporations came into being to
implement local development projects. These special-purpose authorities—
institutions created to accomplish a specific public purpose—were publicly
chartered development institutions run like private corporations, established
specifically to receive a combination of public subsidies and private investment funds.[6] They have often been referred to as public-private corporations
because they thoroughly mixed public resources and powers with private
money and participation, which explains why they easily escape any hint of
partisan politics. Liberal Democratic mayors sit down with Republican business leaders to administer something that seems to be in everyone's interest.

For everyone involved, special authorities are regarded as a pragmatic
solution to a practical problem. Public officials are drawn to special authorities because they allow them to escape the straitjacket of debt limitations
imposed on municipal governments by offloading the costs of development
onto institutions capable of generating their own resources; in this way, general obligation bonds backed by the municipal government can be replaced
by revenue bonds issued by a separate entity. These public-private institutions are generally established through enabling legislation passed by state
legislatures, and they are run by boards appointed by a governor and mayor,
the mayor alone, or some combination of public officials. Because they were
run much like private corporations, they are able to protect their information
and books from public scrutiny.

The examples for three periods in U.S. history lead me to agree with David McDonald's conclusion that "we should not put too much stock in the
value of words themselves." The public-private dualism is often invoked in

debates over the provision of services, but in practice it tends to thoroughly break down. In some ways, this makes things less—not more—complicated because it frees us to focus on the how the local political process actually works, rather than on an abstract and often arcane vocabulary that describes less than it purports to.

## Notes

1. Martin J. Schiesl, *The Politics of Efficiency: Municipal Administration and Reform in America, 1880–1920* (Berkeley: University of California Press, 1977), 80ff.

2. Hazen S. Pingree quoted in Melvin G. Holli, *Reform in Detroit: Hazen S. Pingree and Urban Politics* (New York: Oxford University Press, 1969), 42.

3. Amy Bridges, *Morning Glories: Municipal Reform in the Southwest* (Princeton, N.J.: Princeton University Press, 1997).

4. David Osborne and Ted Gaebler, *Reinventing Government: How the Entrepreneurial Spirit is Transforming the Public Sector* (Reading, Mass.: Addison-Wesley, 1992).

5. Richard M. Daley, "No Pain, No Gain—Or How New York Can Resolve This Crisis and Avert Another; Privatization," *New York Times*, June 16, 1991; Richard M. Daley, "Chicago City Government: Smaller in Size But Greater in Performance," *Business Forum* 19, no. 2 (January 1, 1994): 4; Michael Barone, "The Last Gasp of Liberalism," *U.S. News and World Report* 115, no. 12 (1993): 53.

6. These arrangements are described in Peter K. Eisenger, *The Rise of the Entrepreneurial State: State and Local Economic Development Policy in the United States* (Madison: University of Wisconsin Press, 1988).

# Green Gadgets?

## The Smart-Cities Movement and Urban Environmental Policy

ANTHONY TOWNSEND

*NEW YORK UNIVERSITY*

Most of the world's population are now city dwellers, and mobile, wireless computers outnumber desktops. In an age of urbanization and technological ubiquity, how is the social compact around environmental degradation, science, and policy and planning shifting? What new challenges and what new tools are emerging? This chapter examines three interrelated developments in the smart-cities movement through an environmental policy lens. First, it considers the rapid growth in investment in smart infrastructure designed to improve efficiency, and the impetus provided by global carbon emission reduction efforts. It then looks at shifts in transportation and mobility and potential structural changes in metropolitan land use patterns that may have significant impacts on regional ecosystems. Finally, it examines the implications of distributed sensing for citizen science and debates around urban environmental justice.

## URBANIZATION AND UBIQUITY

### Planet of Cities

It is well understood that we are in the greatest period of city building that humanity may ever know. "The world population will reach a landmark in 2008," United Nations demographers declared in 2007, "for the first time in history the urban population will equal the rural population of the world."[1] Since then every conference—perhaps every single paper—on the future of urbanization begins with this rote observation. Truth be told, the UN was a little overzealous: there's some evidence that the pace of urbanization has slowed, particularly in sub-Saharan Africa, and the 50 percent threshold was not actually crossed until early 2009.[2] Still, economist Paul Romer's observation hits the mark: "In the lifetimes of our children, the urbanization project will be competed. We will have built the system of cities that their descendants will live with forever."[3] And we are well on our way to complete urbanization of the world's population. By 2050, nearly 70 percent of humanity will live in cities.[4] A speculative estimate suggests as many as 90 percent of the world's projected future population of 11 billion will be city dwellers in 2100.[5] The network of built-up areas and connecting infrastructure that supports them will shape the next several centuries of development, if not longer—much as we still live with the geopolitical consequences of the Silk Road, the ports of the Age of Exploration, the railroads of the British Empire, and the U.S. Interstate Highway System.

Yet, even as we make sweeping generalizations about the urban destiny of our civilization, we must recognize the great diversity in the nature of city development across the globe. In the United States—which alone among wealthy countries will add an estimated 90 million new metropolitan inhabitants by 2050—existing metropolitan populations continue to disperse, despite countercurrents of urban revitalization (which is happening at vastly lower densities than historically).[6] Already largely urbanized, Brazil will spend the twenty-first century rebuilding its vast squatter cities, the favelas. In sub-Saharan Africa, where 62 percent of city dwellers live in slums, the urban population is projected to double in population by 2025 (though as noted above, this rate is increasingly the subject of debate). Asian cities, reflecting the tremendous diversity of the largest and most populous continent, are charting a vast range of new forms—from the *desakota* urban-rural sprawl of Indonesia, to Singapore's hyper-managed artificial paradise, to India and China's tandem campaigns to build a hundred "smart cities."

## Connected People and Things

At the precise moment the world became mostly urban, the spread of information and communications technologies (ICTs) passed its own crucial threshold: in 2008, also for the first time, the number of mobile broadband internet subscribers surpassed the number of fixed subscribers. The internet became mostly "untethered"—to borrow a term employed by the U.S. Army in the 1990s as it contemplated the dawning era of telecommunications-enabled mobile urban warfare (and reflecting the reality that "mobile" isn't accurate, since most of us are stationary most of the time when we use our portable devices).[7]

Mobile networks challenge urban planners' intuition about how telecommunications influences travel behavior and land uses. Often, we simplistically assume that by freeing us from wired terminals, mobile phones will allow firms and workers to permanently relocate to rural areas en masse. Yet most evidence points to the opposite. In developing countries, mobile phones have been a powerful enabler of seasonal rural-urban migration (which, not surprisingly, can best be tracked through mobile phone movements recorded by mobile phone companies).[8] Mobiles also reinforce the value of large gathering sites—the essential purpose of cities, after all. For instance, the most robust cellular networks are those that blanket meeting spaces like stadiums and conference centers. Refugees from the Syrian conflict have spread out across Europe with little more than their smartphones in hand.[9] In that sense, mobiles can be seen as a catalyst for density: they get you to the meeting and help you find your friends when you get there.

But there are countercurrents, of course. Mobile networks are also a substrate for sprawl, eliminating the social isolation and opportunity cost of travel by automobile. Not surprisingly, the capital invested in the 285,000 towers that constitute the U.S. cellular grid (about $500 billion, growing at $30–40 billion annually) now rivals that in the U.S. interstate highway system (about $500 billion).[10]

Talking on the go is hardly a new idea—the first mobile phone call was placed in the United States in the 1920s, from the back seat of a specially outfitted automobile in the Philadelphia suburb of Elkins Park. But also in 2008, even as we untethered ourselves from the grid, people become a minority on the internet. Today, there are at least two additional things connected to the internet for every personal device. But forecasts are that by 2020, some 50 billion networked objects will outnumber humans ten to one.

Today, the "internet of things," as these connected objects are collectively known, encompasses a growing range of wearable and portable devices designed for health and fitness applications, home appliances, as well as a growing array of networked automotive systems. As new and retrofitted buildings and urban infrastructure come online, they too will be fitted with embedded sensors and controls. These systems will have tremendous impacts for how cities are managed and planned as businesses, governments, and even citizens tap the pool of observations they create to understand the world, react, and even predict. These "big data" will be an immanent force that pervades and sustains our urban world, and their volume and velocity of production will drown out the entire human web. Consider that one proposed smart city for 200,000 people would produce over 150 times the amount of data contained in all of the 10 billion photos archived on Facebook as of 2013 (about 300 petabytes per year versus Facebook's 1.5 petabyte photo archive).[11] This middling smart city would even put the world's most prolific scientific instrument, the Large Hadron Collider, to shame—that atom-smasher only musters a data flow of about 20 petabytes annually.[12]

## A New Symbiosis

Throughout urban history, the capabilities of ICTs and the size and complexity of cities have advanced hand in hand. City growth drives innovation in information processing tools, and the resulting governance innovations unlock further rounds of urban expansion. In the ancient world, writing supported cities' role as specialized hubs for government, commerce, and religion. In the industrial cities of the nineteenth century, the telegraph, telephone, and mechanical tabulators powered a "control revolution" that coordinated human activity on a previously unimaginable scale.[13] Today, the internet and cellular networks make both urban sprawl and global cities of previously unthinkable size possible—5, 10, or even 20 million people. Without these key technologies, cities would have collapsed under the weight of their own expansion.

As we confront unprecedented urbanization then, in the context of a new revolution in information processing technology, this is the fundamental question: can we employ these tools to manage another round of urban scaling—to megaregions of 40, 50, 75, or 100 million people—while simultaneously delivering a higher standard of living in a more environmentally sustainable and resilient manner?

This is, at its core, what the smart-cities movement is all about.

## From Market to Movement

The term *smart* has entered the global urbanization discourse in the last few years, with little consensus about what it means, what it can contribute to a broader discussion about strategies for improving the urban condition, and its rhetorical limitations. Take, for example, these two statements:

> This is the final phase of industrialization. Everything in your society has to be modernized. Everything has to be smart.[14]

"Smart city" pilot projects are proliferating around the world, bringing together technology companies and cities and towns in public-private partnerships to promote sustainability, conserve energy, reduce costs and meet the needs of citizens who are demanding a reasonable price.[15]

As seen in these quotations, the term *smart* is widely employed by bombastic proponents of corporate-engineered "solutions" to complex urban problems—with a sense of inevitability borrowed from the ICT industry's own mythology.

How "smart" won out over other terms is unclear—it is merely the latest in a lineage dating to the 1970s coined to describe the convergence of cities and ICTs—"wired city," "intelligent city," and "information city" and so on. In 2003, William Mitchell, former dean of the MIT School of Architecture and Planning and an prolific author on the topic, set up at the MIT Media Lab a research group what he named Smart Cities. Adapted by IBM for a multimillion-dollar marketing initiative in 2008 as Smarter Cities, the term seems to have stuck.

Nailing down a definition has been trickier, and scholars have proposed several. A useful one put forth by a major EU-funded effort (the oddly named Fireball Project) weaves technological transformation together with broader goals of citizen empowerment: "A useful definition to start with is to call a city 'smart' when 'investments in human and social capital and traditional (transportation) and modern (ICT-based) infrastructure fuel sustainable economic growth and a high quality of life, with a wise management of natural resources, through participatory government.' . . . To this, the notion of empowerment of citizens and 'democratizing innovation' should be added."[16] Furthermore, the authors tack on to this definition a place-making element, arguing that "the smart city provides the conditions and resources for change. In this sense, the smart city is an urban laboratory, an urban innovation ecosystem, a living lab, an agent of change."[17] In this view, a smart city is defined by the convergence of four elements: human capital development, digital enhancement of infrastructure, citizen engagement through open innovation processes, and a distinct and critical place-based element.

Smart cities, then, are seen as a pragmatic framework for urban management and planning and as highly focused on problem solving. Their broad historic context comes from urbanization and ubiquity. But their immediate context is an economic crisis and the breakdown of global governance. Where old institutions are seen as failing in the face of global challenges, new technologies and insurgent local efforts are seen as viable progressive alternatives. As the Fireball authors put it, the smart city is the engine of transformation, a generator of solutions for wicked problems."[18]

## The Financial Crisis and the Maturing Market

"Black swans" matter.[19] By accident, the 2008 financial crisis was a crucial catalyst for the smart-cities movement, fusing together three trends that came to a boil that year—global urbanization, the mobile internet, and connected things.

While the market was moving in the general direction of smart cities, the financial crisis provoked a sharp and severe cutback in ICT spending by Fortune 500 and multinational corporations—the bread-and-butter customers of technology vendors such as IBM, Cisco, and Oracle. Aside from travel, ICT capital spending was one of the easiest places to trim and stockpile cash for what looked at the time to be a very volatile and extended, and potentially catastrophic, period of economic and financial uncertainty.

At the same time, however, government stimulus spending began to ramp up in the United States, Europe, and East Asia. Urban infrastructure represented the most promising opportunity for technology vendors to capture post-crisis stimulus spending. One widely circulated forecast, published in 2007 by consultancy Booz Allen Hamilton, claimed that global infrastructure needs would top $1.5 trillion annually for the next twenty-five years—just shy of 3 percent of global GDP. According to the Urban Land Institute, a real estate industry think tank, the United States alone needed to spend $2 trillion to repair and rebuild its decaying infrastructure.[20]

The bulk of infrastructure spending—97 percent—will be on conventional materials like asphalt and steel. But as much as 3 percent could go to ICT, which sets an upped bound for spending on the digital aspects of smart-city solutions. This figure is remarkably constant; either looking at the global scale (e.g., by comparing market forecasts for smart infrastructure to total infrastructure) or a large development project (e.g., Songdo City in South Korea, whose ICT business strategist reports 2.9 percent), or a single building (which can be gleaned from a variety of trade publications).

Smart-city ICT comes in three layers, according to engineering consultancy Arup: instrumentation that collects data throughout the city; urban informatics systems that process the signals; and an urban information architecture, or set of management practices and business processes, to put the results to use. Andrew Comer, a partner at construction engineering firm Buro Happold explains the cocktail-party math: "If you project that figure into the future, multiply it by a fairly conservative estimate of the construction costs involved, and take a relatively small percentage of that for high-technology infrastructure, it's trillions of dollars. If these hi-tech companies can capture parts of this market, they have a twenty to thirty year period of insatiable growth." Thus, smart cities promise to be a cash cow for the technology industry, chalking up some $100 billion in potential revenues over the next decade. And that's even before the management consulting fees—for, as Arup argued in 2010, "the smart city is so different in essence to the 20th century city that the governance models and organisational frameworks themselves must evolve."[21]

By 2011, even conglomerates like Siemens and GE had turned their attention to the smart-cities market, sensing even greater potential than the ICT niche that IBM and Cisco had unearthed. As Peter Löscher, CEO of Siemens put it, "this is a huge, huge opportunity." Yet, in the years since 2008, despite thousands of conferences, pilot projects, and other campaigns, the ambitions of these firms have largely been unrealized. As the *Economist* reported in 2013, "many cities lack the necessary resources for the more ambitious dreams of city planners. Companies such as Cisco, IBM and Siemens are all eager to sell them systems. 'None has met its revenue targets,' says a smart-city expert at a big consultancy. A new 'infrastructure and cities' division at Siemens has the lowest profit margin of all of Siemens's big businesses."[22] The reasons for inflated expectations are many but largely have to do with misperceptions about the decision-making processes of local governments, a lack of easily repurposable business models, and a poor job selling the value of investments to actual end users—the citizens themselves. But despite the setbacks of these old-line tech giants, the smart-cities market has continued to expand, mature, and evolve in a number of ways that suggest its long-term viability.

This is most clearly seen in the exponentially expanding size and scope of the smart-cities market forecasts. One widely noted study, published in 2011 by Colorado-based Pike Research (now part of Navigant) pegged the total market at $100 billion in annual sales globally by 2020.[23] But soon after, at the behest of the U.K. government, Arup produced a new forecast, which expanded the range of services, more than quadrupling the market to $408 billion per year by 2020.[24] Just over twelve months later, consultancy Frost & Sullivan in its own estimate again quadrupled the pie to $1.56 trillion.[25]

What is the significance of these ballooning forecasts? Partly it reflects the growing expectations among an expanding array of stakeholders—banking on the smart-city market to expand is not just IBM, but the U.K. government as well, as part of its export-led economic growth policy. Also, definitions of the sector are expanding (notably from the Pike to the Arup forecast) to include a larger range of value-added services riding on top of smart infrastructure, recognizing where the true nexus of innovation lies. Finally, there is a growing sense of the massive "dark-matter" cloud of start-ups and SMEs moving into the market and developing new niches with considerable potential—as seen in networks like Urban.Us and CityMart, which are trying to challenge traditional geographic obstacles to city-vendor procurement and startup-investor relationships and to help fledging firms expand globally beyond their initial launch cities.

But perhaps far more significantly, these forecasts are beginning to reflect the arrival of the big consumer-facing ICT companies in the smart-city market—Google, Apple, Intel, and Microsoft—all of which are now forming groups, developing strategies, making acquisitions, and launching initiatives in this space. (Full disclosure: I am a consultant to Sidewalk Labs, of which Google is a major investor, and I have previously consulted for Intel). Given that IBM and Cisco may have failed to capture citizens' imagination because they lacked experience with consumers, this could signal a crucial development.

## The Political Economy of Smart Cities

So far, we have largely looked at the corporate agenda for smart cities, yet as Plato reminds us in *The Republic*, the city is and has always been a contested social and economic space: "For indeed any city, however small, is in fact divided into two, one the city of the poor, the other of the rich; these are at war with one another."[26] For every potential productivity or efficiency gain, smart technologies present a redistributive risk. Considerable serious debate is now underway, for instance, about the possibility of mass unemployment as intelligent systems are widely deployed in the coming decades, and the potential for catastrophic impacts on income and wealth distribution.[27] Several efforts to map the political economy of smart cities have been widely circulated, including the author's.[28] These seek to shift the locus of attention from the "what" of smart systems—the technologies and their applications—to the "why" and "how." The more successful ones, such as Elie Cosgrave's doctoral thesis on Bristol's smart-city policy framework in England, succeed by dissecting competing interests around specific projects in communities.

But even as global technology companies have dominated discussions about smart cities over the last decade, a parallel grassroots movement has coalesced. To use a computing metaphor: if industry has produced a mainframe vision of a smart city, the alternative is something akin to the personal computer: inexpensive and decentralized. Three big shifts in technology are enabling this shift. First, as already mentioned, computing has moved off the desktop. By 2011, sales of personal computers were flat, while smartphones and tablets sold in record numbers. These devices not only decentralize computing power from large organizations into the hands of everyday people, they also embed it in everyday urban spaces, spurring new ideas about potential uses. Second, the shift from fixed to untethered communications is pushing information technology into every crevice of the city. Third, cloud computing has decoupled information processing from place, enabling supercomputing power to be accessed from any device, anytime, anywhere—including our pockets. These raw materials provide a vastly expanded array of basic components for entrepreneurs, tinkerers, and media artists to develop novel responses to urban challenges—giving rise to services as varied as Uber (for e-hailing rides), SeeClickFix (for local information), and HandUp (for donating to homeless individuals). Hal Varian, Google's chief economist, has likened the situation to the early industrial era, when standardized machine parts spurred a global frenzy of "combinatorial innovation."[29] Where the corporate smart city primarily seeks to control, optimize, and make efficient, the bottom-up version also aspires to enhance access, sociability, transparency, and entertainment.

What of city government then? What is its role in this? As I wrote in 2013, it seemed a battle was brewing over the soul of the smart city: "Everywhere that industry attempts to impose its vision of clean, computed, centrally managed order, [civic hackers] propose messy, decentralized, and democratic alternatives. It's only a matter of time before they come to blows."[30] While they have rebuffed the most audacious visions of industry, city governments have not yet really embraced a fully citizen-powered vision of the smart city either. For now, they seem to be trying to balance interests, and identify sustainable strategies for innovation over the long term.

They are doing this through two primary means: creating new leadership positions and developing digital master plans. New leadership positions such as chief innovation officers, chief technology officers, chief data officers, and chief digital officers, have given cities the ability to coordinate and elevate technology policy and planning within city government, and leverage external resources in the private sector, universities, and the philanthropic community. Digital master plans represent a new comprehensive, long-range urban planning activity, seeking to develop a vision and road map for investments in ICTs that align with citywide policy.[31]

The political economy of the smart city is still in flux, and alliances and alignments of course vary from place to place—the relationship between industry and city government runs from hot to cold, and the same for civic hacker groups, as well. Meanwhile, universities are moving en masse to position themselves as key players through the establishment of urban science and urban informatics centers and so-called living labs for smart-city engineering.[32]

## SMART CITIES AND THE ENVIRONMENT

During the Progressive Era, widespread recognition of the threats to public health presented by overcrowding and poor sanitation in U.S. cities led to the launch of numerous reform programs. These efforts improved sanitary conditions through improvements in water and sewer infrastructure and housing stocks. At the same time, conservationists achieved a consensus around the need to prevent further damage and depletion of natural resources from human settlement and industrial activity.

As the environmental movement matured in the postwar period, new scientific evidence gave rise to a loose compact of interests, which played an increasing role in spurring nations and regions to address the effects and roots causes of environmental degradation. Previously, externalities from industrial production could be ignored, as those costs could be off-loaded to surrounding neighborhoods, downstream residents, or downwind lakes. But as suburban sprawl brought city and countryside into more direct contact, these distinctions began to break down.

Increasingly, this compact (especially at its scientific roots in the case of climate change) is being attacked, but is it unraveling? As they provide new tools for monitoring, regulating, and managing urban environments, to what extent does the smart-cities movement reinvigorate the public debate over the social compact on environmental sustainability and the protection of the larger society?

We turn now to three themes where the smart-cities movement is directly engaging structural underpinnings of the urban environmental compact, also posing a number of questions for further discussion and research. These themes are infrastructural complexity and efficiency, transportation innovation, and citizen science.

### Infrastructural Complexity and Efficiency

One of the key engineering challenges of future cities is infrastructural complexity. Delivering responsive, high-quality urban services requires careful integration of many different networked resources in a carefully synchronized fashion. For instance, mass deployment of electric vehicles will require new approaches to balancing the flow of vehicles on road networks as well as the flow of energy on power grids, and the interactions between the two dynamic systems. As social demands for reliability and resilience increase, increasingly distributed points of generation and distribution will further complicate matters. Meanwhile, the liberating impacts of ICTs on individuals and organizations—breaking down traditional schedules and travel routes—are creating more differentiated infrastructure usage patterns, further complicating the picture.

Coping with the complexity of infrastructure itself, and the rapidly changing and increasingly dynamic patterns of use, will require new approaches from operators. Three possibilities present themselves.

First, even as complexity is a challenge, it can also be a tool. By engineering entire systems, we can exploit new synergies, such as cogeneration, which uses waste heat from industrial processes to produce electricity. This well-established approach is being developed in many efforts, but it is largely incremental in the gains it presents.

Second, new sensory capabilities of smart cities, when linked to predictive computer models, can allow for infrastructure to be managed in a far more optimized fashion than before. For instance, renewable energy sources such as solar present a particularly difficult problem given the unpredictability of the weather and the high cost of building storage for cloudy days. But, as researchers at the National Center for Atmospheric Research and Xcel Energy in Boulder, Colorado, have shown, highly accurate solar forecasts can be used to balance supply and demand in real time over a wide area. In one experiment, the group briefly supplied 60 percent of the state's power needs exclusively from solar.[33] This is an example of what we might call a super-intelligent city, where machine intelligence performs analytical and allocation functions largely beyond the scope of possible human understanding (but with human oversight, at least for now). It is, essentially, a fly-by-wire city. Take away the computers and it falls apart. For a sneak preview of this in practice, we need only look at some of the more recent innovations in active structural control, which operate in much the same way.

An alternative approach, which addresses the lack of transparency inherent in the previous example (assuming that the model uses machine learning, it is probably illegible) is what is called human task routing. Here the idea is to assemble a large group of human beings online to disaggregate portions of a large, complex task into smaller, discrete tasks that can be more easily completed and then to reassemble the completed work into a finished product. We might imagine this being used to analyze data about energy flows in a city, analyze signals intelligence for counterterrorism efforts, or look for signs of socioeconomic distress in data collected at city schools. Such approaches are currently employed in a number of crowdsourced online work platforms such as ODesk, Mobileworks, and Amara for tasks like market research, writing documents, transcription, and translation.[34]

A third approach to infrastructural complexity and efficiency is simply behavior change—trying to "nudge" people (to use Thaler and Sunstein's 2008 term) to reduce burdens on infrastructure. This raises some of the most intriguing possibilities because we start to enter a world where the market-based innovations that we have seen in telecommunications are unleashed on the consumer energy sector. In the 1980s, when digitization of the phone system allowed more calls to be squeezed onto the same trunk lines, it also put intelligence in the network. Creating new services like call waiting, voice mail, and caller ID was then simply a matter of writing new switching software.[35] Proponents of smart power grids expect a similar wave of innovation in energy services. Start-up firms could audit and manage home electricity use in return for a small cut of the energy bill reduction. Automating that process would be advantageous in a world where Siemens forecasts that electricity prices could change as often as every fifteen minutes.[36] Smart grids could also map our social networks to the production, distribution, and consumption of electricity. Eric Paulos of the University of California, Berkeley, proposes using sensors to document how, where, and by whom energy is generated and making this information available during transactions. Such metadata could enable markets for power around any number of causes, interests, or goals. Today, power suppliers largely compete on price and on carbon footprint. A smart grid could allow the data about electricity to become as valuable as the power itself, and such data could enable better decisions about how we use electricity.[37]

Smart-city innovations in efficiency, and the infrastructure complexity they will manage and require be put in place to achieve them, raise many questions about environmental compact.

- How will the public perceive the complex cause-and-effect relationships within these systems and the environmental outcomes they produce?
- How will the roles of software and algorithms be made more transparent? How can the assumptions of model builders be scrutinized and their implications examined?
- What is the role of human oversight in the automation of urban infrastructure systems?

- What ethical issues are involved in choosing between automating efficient behaviors and seeking to induce behavior change?

### Transportation Innovation

The smart-cities movement is also having a more direct impact on the public debate around the social compact on environmental sustainability in transportation innovation.

While enormous changes have occurred in urban U.S. businesses, governments, and society in the last 25 years, little has changed in transportation. One could make the case that the way we get around—from the technology, to the business models, to the regulatory schemes—has not changed in 75 years (for surface transportation) to 125 years or more (for rail and ferry transit).

Yet in the last several years we have seen the introduction of a string of innovations, almost exclusively privately initiated, that are dramatically changing transportation business models, challenging existing regulatory schemes head-on, and most importantly, portending substantial long-term shifts in travel patterns and land use in our inner cities and larger metropolitan areas in coming years—shifts that could have both profound positive and negative impacts on regional ecosystems. Thousands of new digital technologies and services have come to market in recent years that are turning transportation from a bricks-and-mortar business into an information-based and informatics-based activity.

Disruption is happening throughout the value chain, as in the following examples.

- Infrastructure networks: adaptive traffic signaling, electronic road pricing
- Vehicles: autonomous vehicles, programmable vehicle performance
- Business models: car sharing, ride sharing
- Interfaces: crowdsourced traffic reporting, multi-model integration

The result of all this investment and innovation is that city dwellers are increasingly dependent on an array of digital services and technologies to make and manage travel choices, and often also dependent on them to actually take the trip. These services are having real impacts on travel behavior, changing why, when, where, and how people take journeys to work, home, and other locations and activities. They are changing both the supply and the demand sides of the travel equation.

Ironically, while transportation planners are mostly unaware of the interactions between new ICTs and travel behavior, and their implications for future land use needs, some start-ups are tackling this head-on. For instance, the carpooling service Zimride, launched at the University of California, Berkeley, but later deployed for two large music festivals (Coachella and Bonaroo), is a platform for large venue and facility operators to coordinate and incentivize carpooling. Over the long run, services like Zimride could allow large amounts of land now tied up for parking to be freed for development, potentially creating a virtuous circle of densification that could create greater demand for transit.

Transportation planning is only slowly waking up to these developments. Internal debates in the field remain focused on infrastructure and urban form rather than on the direct behavioral impacts of these new technologies. As a result, these high-value, high-impact innovations in transportation are coming from the private sector with little coordination or planning. And their collective impact and potential unintended consequences are not being adequately explored.

Take, for instance, the conflicts between Uber and local regulators. It is clear that the conflicts between innovators and regulators that we are seeing now are merely suggestive of much larger challenges to come. These are just the initial skirmishes in much bigger conflicts that will arise over how transportation systems will work in twenty-first-century cities, and over the roles and relationships between public- and private-sector providers. The rapid private-sector innovation-driven shift in transportation—which I call reprogramming mobility—has profound consequences for the environmental compact in the United States, as it ties together the two most significant environmental choices most U.S. households make: their choice of residence and their mode of commuting. Some questions include the following.

- How can transportation planners understand, forecast, and explain alternative transportation futures to communities?
- What kinds of narratives can create compelling linkages between individual transportation choice architectures on the one hand and community goals and visions and global environmental impacts on the other?
- What are the actual trade-offs among the three assets of land use, transportation, and ICTs? What substitutes and what complements? What kinds of new, more sustainable designs and forms are possible (e.g., televillages, or whatever is the next version of them—such as the

Washington, D.C., developer who secured a zoning change to eliminate a required parking deck by giving every resident a bike share
membership)?

### Citizen Science

In 1976, when Steve Jobs and Steve Wozniak demonstrated the Apple-1 pro-
totype at the Homebrew Computer Club in Palo Alto, California, just down
the road from Menlo Park (where the more radical People's Computer Company, another user group, gathered), the electronics community in Northern
California was abuzz with the potential of democratized computing power.
Today, the same urges that set off that revolution can be felt within the networks of inventors, entrepreneurs, tinkerers, and researchers exploring the
potential of connected objects, environments, buildings, and cities. And as
the ability to cheaply and quickly deploy sensors in the city meets up with the
long-established traditions of citizen science developed in fields as varied as
astronomy and ornithology, the smart-cities movement is poised to breathe
new energy into the urban environmental justice movement.

In recent years, the internet has allowed scientists to engage ever-larger
groups of amateurs in collecting and analyzing data, in much the same way
that meteorologists have long collected weather and climate data from a
distributed network of volunteer-maintained instruments and stations. Amateurs have made important discoveries in many areas of science, such as
astronomy, by analyzing large sets of data. They have also played a major
role in formulating research questions as well, such as the growing interest
in rare diseases, which were largely ignored until victims could find each
other, share information, and organize online.

But citizens aren't waiting for universities to launch their own research.
Urban environmental sensing is a particularly intense area of citizen-driven
scientific data collection. In Paris, for instance, the internet think tank
Fing (Foundation Internet Nouvelle Génération) developed a wristwatch
for measuring street-level ozone. In a demonstration involving a hundred
bicyclists riding in a single neighborhood, volunteers were able to create a
finely detailed air pollution map that dramatically surpassed the government's sparse network of just ten stations across the entire city. At MIT's
SENSEable City Laboratory, researchers took some rudimentary GPS-en-
abled phones, glued them to various pieces of rubbish and threw them away.
Within days, they had generated a map of the removal chain, illuminating
the secret journeys of our waste. In New York, a group calling itself Pub-

lic Laboratory builds inexpensive sensors that alert citizens to situations during thunderstorms when the city's storm-water drains overflow into its sewage system, causing coastal discharge of human waste. The intent is that ambient displays in homes would spur people to refrain from flushing toilets during these events, thus reducing the flow of raw sewage into waterways.

As mentioned previously, universities are seizing the chance to stake out new territory in smart cities. Just since about 2010, a vast array of new academic and nonprofit institutions have been established to develop and exploit these new data streams to advance human understanding and improve the management of cities. From New York University's Center for Urban Science and Progress to the University of Chicago's Urban Center for Computation and Data to the Intel Collaborative Research Institute for Sustainable and Connected Cities in London, it has become clear that this is going to be a major global research theme, one with considerable potential impact across a huge range of policy arenas.

Not surprisingly, many of the new urban science labs—including MIT's SENSEable City Lab and NYU's Center for Urban Science and Progress— are directly engaging with these kinds of citizen urban science efforts. This makes sense, since the nature and scale of the subject of interest (cities) almost demand a strategy of leveraging citizens as extensions of the university's capacities.

More important, however, is that including citizens in research makes it potentially more likely that they will welcome the results of the research as valid and accept their use in the design of new interventions. Engaging citizen science may represent a strategy for making this wave of urban science, and its application in the public sector, significantly less technocratic than what we have seen in the past, and make the research itself into an act of civic engagement. Open data will play a crucial catalyzing role in those collaborations.

Citizen urban science raises a bewildering number of questions about the environmental compact, including these two:

- Will citizen urban science focus mostly on augmenting professional data gathering, filling in gaps, or creating alternative narratives that challenge official data?
- What is the role of open data platforms in facilitating collaborations between citizens, universities, and city governments in urban research?

## IMPLICATIONS FOR PLANNING RESEARCH

We have looked at the rise of the smart-cities movement and its emerging intersections with urban environmental policy in three areas: infrastructural complexity, transportation innovation, and citizen science. Further elaboration on the potential for citizen science to inform planning research is warranted, and a cautionary tale about the overall prospects of the smart-cities movement to achieve meaningful long-term environmental results.

### Citizen Urban Science and Future Collaboration

The nature of urban research appears to be changing rapidly. Universities around the world are bringing online a massive new infrastructure for data-driven urban research in the coming decades—an investment that could surpass $2.5 billion by 2030. But the new urban science, as many are calling this movement, has not yet defined how it intends to engage or empower non-professionals in the research process—a glaring omission in an age in which new digital platforms are unleashing the power of mass participation in so many other areas of the economy, governance, and intellectual and political life.[38] While there is much talk of the importance of citizens in these efforts as beneficiaries of research effort, their envisioned role in the research process is far less clear. Predominantly, these efforts envision future urban research as a tripartite collaboration of university, city government, and private sector firms. But will this new intellectual venture be an inclusive endeavor? What role is there for the growing ranks of increasingly well-equipped and well-informed citizen volunteers and amateur investigators to work alongside professional scientists? How are researchers, activists, and city governments exploring that potential today? Finally, what can be done to encourage and accelerate experimentation?[39]

Citizen science has thrived in recent years as these changes have unfolded. While amateurs have long played important roles in many fields, from astronomy to meteorology, the Web has lowered the cost and expanded the range of collaborative activities with professional scientists. For instance, amateurs now routinely participate not only in the analysis of large data sets, but in so doing help train computer software to perform the same tasks. There is so much citizen science happening now that the practice itself is becoming a field of academic inquiry itself—in early 2015 the prestigious journal *Bioscience* called for the recognition of "research on citizen science as a distinct discipline."[40]

Urban research is changing quickly, but its relationship with citizen science will inevitably become deeply complex and multifaceted, and controversial. That's because not only is citizen science a necessary key to improving the science of cities, it is a tool for making the case that the results of such research are to be trusted when applied in urban governance. Citizen science can provide the ground truth necessary to trust the synoptic urban sensing tools being used in urban science. Our operating hypothesis is threefold. First, we expect that citizen urban science will become an increasingly important strategy within the urban science movement—for doing better science, by creating larger and more detailed data sets. Second, it will be used to render the pursuit of science less technocratic, by giving citizens a stake in data gathering, analysis, application of results, and even setting parts of the research agenda. Third, it will create legitimacy to apply new knowledge in the real world, by creating sustained engagement between researchers and partners in local governments for tech transfer.

The way that citizen urban science evolves will both shape and be shaped by the legacy of the environmental justice movement over the last half-century, which demonstrated how citizen urban science can have major lasting impacts on urban policy and planning, and the lives of people and groups in urban communities. Environmental justice itself grew directly out of the civil-rights struggle—in 1968 Martin Luther King Jr. fought on behalf of black sanitation workers in Memphis.[41] The environmental justice movement coalesced in the 1970s and 1980s through activist efforts, which focused attention on the systematic biases and shortcomings of environmental risk assessment practices in the United States—especially around urban air pollution impacts of siting decisions for highly noxious public facilities such as incinerators, trash transfer stations, and waste treatment plants.

In the 1990s, the movement began to trigger reforms on urban environmental policy at the federal level. Robert Bullard's landmark report *Dumping in Dixie: Race, Class, and Environmental Quality* (1990) led directly to the Clinton administration's 1994 executive order mandating environmental justice reviews in the conduct of federal government operations.[42] But despite its origins in a movement based on its appeal to human rights, ethics, and fairness, data and quantitative evidence have been critical to building support and a record of victories for the movement. Citizen- and activist-collected data have been used to win cases on the behalf of communities unfairly targeted as hosts for threats to public health, such as nuclear-waste disposal and industrial facilities.[43] Such data were used to contest the federal government's own assessment tools, which had become so institutionalized that their weaknesses were called an open secret.[44]

Although environmental justice had a contentious relationship in the past with professional science—the movement generally viewed traditional science as cold and detached, and unwilling or unable to incorporate social factors into environmental hazard assessment, whereas the scientists saw environmental justice advocates as unorganized and emotional—the movement still wielded scientific data and methods to serve its own ends with great prowess and effectiveness. Evidence-based campaigns have been effective in policy circles at the federal level, bringing change to the ways the EPA conducts environmental assessments as well as leading to the creation of the Office of Environmental Justice, but these efforts still face challenges. Despite the massive amount of citizen-collected data the movement has produced, very little of it has been utilized in formal scientific research, where it is still often viewed with extreme skepticism.[45]

Today's efforts to link environmental concerns with citizen cover a broad spectrum of models for bringing together citizens, academic researchers, and government agencies to do urban research. A recent paper looks at three case studies:

- Chicago's Array of Things: a large-scale urban environmental sensor network blanketing the downtown Loop, established to provide a test bed for university research and citizen engagement.
- Amsterdam's Smart-Citizens Lab: a training and prototyping facility in Amsterdam that seeks to develop a corps of citizen scientists to deploy and maintain sensors throughout the city.
- New York City's Trees Count!: a crowdsourced effort to conduct a decennial census of street trees to support ongoing planning and operations, and potential future research.[46]

These early efforts to mobilize citizens to advance the collection, analysis and application of urban data in cities highlight both the promise and the nascent nature of citizen urban science today. Although citizen science has spread broadly around the globe and garnered attention from national policy makers, this movement is only slowly gaining traction at the city level.[47] As these projects and others like them progress, the utility of citizen generated data is substantial. Yet further efforts are necessary to organize and direct the trajectory of citizen urban science for it to have the transformative impact demonstrated by the environmental justice movement.

Three emerging nodes of collaboration that should be targeted for further research and support in the immediate future—shared sensing infrastructure, open data, and networked social capital.

SHARED SENSING INFRASTRUCTURE:    Each of these efforts began with research and development of a new instrument for data collection—the Array of Things sensor pod, the Smart Citizen Kit, and the tablet app used by Trees Count! This is counterintuitive, because advocates of participatory digital urbanism routinely point to mass ownership of smartphones as a fundamental enabler of citizen urban science—yet each of the projects saw the need to invest considerable resources and time in deploying a new, customized data collection platform. A key question going forward is whether increasing fragmentation of infrastructure is expected or desirable, or if, as Array of Things and Smart Citizen Kit implicitly aspire, there is an opportunity to colocate most of the required sensors for a portfolio of efforts, organizations, and projects on a single physical infrastructure. If this is technically feasible, how can it be made financially and institutionally feasible? (For instance, what happens when conflicts over sensor requirements occur?)

OPEN DATA:    The open-data movement has demonstrated how sharing of information without restrictions can, as Code for America founder Jennifer Pahlka describes it, "allow us to collaborate without talking about it."[48] However, significant obstacles inhibit realizing the full potential of open data to catalyze and accelerate citizen urban science. As we saw in environmental justice, government officials and even academic researchers are often skeptical of the quality and bias of citizen-generated data. Even where they are collected, and pressing policy issues exist, they are likely to be ignored. Citizen advocacy groups may balk at sharing data that could be used to frame a case against their preferred course of action. Researchers, while increasingly being pressured to open research data for review and subsequent use, have powerful incentives to hoard valuable research data. Future research should probe further into the value chains that develop and can be developed around urban sensor data, and the way open sharing can help accumulate and distribute that value in equitable and productive flows. We expect that this will require deep ethnographic and managerial types of studies.

NETWORKED SOCIAL CAPITAL:    The key to understanding and enabling these value chains will be focused effort on catalyzing and cultivating the networked social capital that gives rise to and sustains citizen urban science undertakings. Each of these cases addresses this node of collaboration in a substantial way— the Array of Things has created a dense network of institutional partnerships, the Smart Citizens Lab is focused on recruiting and training a grassroots cadre of citizen-scientists, and Trees Count! seeks to build an army of volunteers who can be mobilized in times of need by government to provide a public service. Yet important questions remain: How can these models be made replicable? How do they complement or compete with each other? What models are best suited to which aspirations of citizen urban science—for example, collection of scientific data, issue advocacy and policy change, community and economic development?

### Thinking about the Unthinkable

There is no doubt that smart cities are a key area of concern for urban planning and that urban environmental monitoring is a key application area at the highest levels of federal policymaking—statements to this effect by key Obama administration officials at smart-city events in 2015 make this clear.[49] And there are competing visions for how to accomplish this—through coordinated, centralized, city-led, and corporate-enabled deployment of comprehensive sensing grids, or through more citizen-driven, distributed frameworks. There is every reason to believe that at least one of these approaches might work, both could work independently, or they might even complement each other in a new beautiful synergy—in fact, that wouldn't be all that different from how the internet and the World Wide Web has worked out (with a few caveats).

But I would be remiss as a forecaster if I didn't paint a somewhat darker picture of what might lie ahead. For we need to approach smart cities with skepticism, to think about the worst that could happen, and how we might face it. For the implicit assumption in nearly all framings of the smart-cities concept is that they will be more efficient and better for the environment than contemporary urbanization frameworks. But there are many scenarios, eminently plausible, where this is a false assumption. Let us close by considering a few.

First, smart technology might not deliver enough efficiency. The improvement needed to stabilize carbon dioxide emissions are "neither trivial nor impossible," according to a 2007 United Nations Foundation report. But they are certainly not a sure thing. In the worst case, more efficient smart infrastructure will actually work to hold down the price of energy and stimulate even more consumption—what economists call the "rebound effect."[50]

Second, smart technology might turn out to be less effective in curbing energy use, yet highly effective for reducing traffic congestion and fighting crime. Although cities in developed nations would become more appealing places to live as the quality of life improved, also indirectly reducing energy consumption by drawing people back from the suburbs to denser communities, in the developing world it could accelerate the growth of megacities powered by today's dirty energy technologies. That would be an economic success story of epic proportion but a global ecological disaster. Imagine a smart Johannesburg suddenly free of crime and booming, absorbing millions of migrants from sub-Saharan Africa into a ramshackle infrastructure of dirty minibuses and smoky coal- and dung-fueled stoves.

A third doomsday story goes like this: we do crack the code of sustainable design and bring the needed technologies to market—but not in time. Even in Singapore, with its long and proven tradition of technocratic planning, smart-infrastructure projects move at a snail's pace; digitization of the nation-state's congestion toll system was twelve years in the making, finally implemented in 1998.

A fourth possibility is economic stagnation. If the malaise of the developing world is too much growth, for the rich cities of the global north it may be too little. If, as many economists now suspect, smart technology cannot improve our productivity, we might not be able to pay for further improvements in energy efficiency.

In a final unthinkable future, the wealthy fall back on smart technology to retreat to gated enclaves, sustained by captured resources managed solely for their own benefit. This is already the norm across much of the developing world, where the poor have less access to clean water, healthy food, and basic sanitation, and pay vastly higher prices for them when they do. As competition for natural resources heats up over the next century, and the impacts of climate change disrupt supplies, the rich may be able to wall themselves off from the consequences of their own overconsumption. Instead of making cities more resilient to the challenges of rapid growth and climate change, smart technology could limit the ability of poor and vulnerable communities to adapt.

## Notes

1. "World Urbanization Prospects: The 2007 Revision," United Nations, Department of Economic and Social Affairs, Population Division—Population Estimates and Projections Section, New York, February 26, 2008, 1.

2. "World Urbanization Prospects: The 2009 Revision," (New York: United Nations, Department of Economic and Social Affairs, Population Division—Population Estimates and Projections Section, New York, March 2010, 1.

3. Paul Romer, "Charter Cities." Accessed April 11, 2016. http://econ.as.nyu.edu/docs/IO/22933/Romer1_02132012.pdf

4. "World Urbanization Prospects: The 2011 Revision," United Nations, Department of Economic and Social Affairs, Population Division—Population Estimates and Projections Section, New York, March 2012, 1.

5. Author's calculation based on global population forecast in *The 2010 Revision of World Population Prospects* and urbanization forecast of 70 to 80 percent in Shlomo Angel, *Planet of Cities* (Cambridge, Mass.: Lincoln Institute of Land Policy, 2012).

6. IHS Global Insight, "U.S. Metro Economies: Outlook—Gross Metropolitan Product, and Critical Role of Transportation Infrastructure," United States Conference of Mayors, 2012, accessed August 20, 2015, at http://usmayors.org/metroeconomies/0712/FullReport.pdf.

7. D. A. Hall, "Tactical Internet System Architecture for Task Force XXI," *IEEE*, 1996, 219–30, doi:10.1109/TCC.1996.561089.

8. Amy Wesolowski and Nathan Eagle, "Inferring Human Dynamics in Slums Using Mobile Phone Data," Working Paper, Santa Fe Institute, accessed August 20, 2015, at http://www.santafe.edu/media/cms_page_media/264/AmyWesolowskiREU FinalPaper.pdf.

9. Matthew Brunwasser, "A 21st-Century Migrant's Essentials: Food, Shelter, Smartphone," *New York Times*, August 25, 2015.

10. "U.S. Wireless Quick Facts," Cellular Telecommunications Industry Association, accessed February 3, 2013, at http://www.ctia.org/consumer_info/index.cfm/AI D/10323; Massoud Amin, "North American Electricity Infrastructure: System Security, Quality, Reliability, Availability, and Efficiency Challenges and their Societal Impacts," in *Continuing Crises in National Transmission Infrastructure: Impacts and Options for Modernization*, National Science Foundation (NSF), June 2004, 1; "CTIA Semi-Annual Wireless Industry Survey," Cellular Telecommunications Industry Association, Washington, D.C., 2012, accessed September 1, 2015, at http://www.ctia.org/your-wireless-life/how-wireless-works/annual-wireless-industry-survey.

11. Rich Miller, "Facebook Hosts 10 Billion Photos," Data Center Knowledge, accessed July 30, 2015, at http://www.datacenterknowledge.com/archives/2008/10/15/facebook-hosts-10-billion-photos/.

12. "Living PlanIT—PlanIT Valley—A Smart and Connected City for Portugal," accessed July 26, 2015, at http://www.living-planit.com

13. Charles Perrow, *Normal Accidents: Living with High-Risk Technologies*, rev. ed. (Princeton, N.J.: Princeton University Press, 1999 [1984]).

14. Steve Hamm, "Live Blogging from Smarter Cities Rio: Day 1," *Building a Smarter Planet: A Smarter Planet Blog*, November 9, 2011, accessed January 25, 2011, at http://asmarterplanet.com/blog/2011/11/live-blogging-from-smarter-cities-rio-day-1.html.

15. "World Economic Forum Annual Meeting 2012: The Great Transformation: Shaping New Models," World Economic Forum, Davos-Klosters, Switzerland, 2012, 25, accessed June 18, 2015, at http://www3.weforum.org/docs/AM12/WEF_AM12_Report .pdf.

16. Hans Schaffers, Nicos Komninos, Marc Pallot, et al., "Smart Cities as Innovation Systems Sustained by the Future Internet," technical report 2012, URENIO Research

Unit, Thessaloniki, Greece, 2012, 5, accessed at http://www.urenio.org/wp-content/uploads/2012/04/2012-FIREBALL-White-Paper-Final.pdf.

17. Ibid., 6.

18. Ibid., 57.

19. Nicholas Nassim Taleb, *The Black Swan: The Impact of the Highly Improbable* (New York: Random House, 2007).

20. Jonathan D. Miller, "Infrastructure 2011: A Strategic Priority," Urban Land Institute and Ernst & Young, 2011, accessed September 1, 2015, at http://www.uli.org/ResearchAndPublications/%7E/media/Documents/ResearchAndPublications/Reports/Infrastructure/Infrastructure2011.ashx.

21. Andrew Comer and Kerwin Datu, "Can You Have a Private City? The Political Implications of 'Smart City' Technology," *Global Urbanist*, last modified February 11, 2011, http:// globalurbanist.com/2011/02/17/can-you-have-a-private-city-the-political-implications-of- smart-city-technology; "Smart Cities: Transforming the 21st Century City via the Creative Use of Technology," Arup, last modified September 1, 2010, 10, accessed September 14, 2015, at http://www.arup.com/Publications/Smart_Cities.aspx.

22. "The Multiplexed Metropolis," *Economist*, September 7, 2013, accessed July 23, 2015 at http://www.economist.com/news/briefing/21585002-enthusiasts-think-data-services-can-change-cities-century-much-electricity.

23. "Smart Cities: Intelligent Information and Communications Technology Infrastructure in the Government, Buildings, Transport, and Utility Domains," Pike Research, online report, 2011, no longer available.

24. "The Smart City Market: Opportunities for the UK," research paper, Department for Business Innovation and Skills, and ARUP, London, 2013.

25. "Frost & Sullivan: Global Smart Cities Market to Reach US$1.56 Trillion by 2020," Frost & Sullivan, accessed Jannuary 25, 2011, at http://ww2.frost.com/news/press-releases/frost-sullivan-global-smart-cities-market-reach-us156-trillion-2020/.

26. Plato, *The Republic*, Internet Classics Archive, accessed April 11, 2016, at http://classics.mit.edu/Plato/republic.5.iv.html.

27. For instance, see Erik Brynjolfsson and Andrew McAfee, *The Second Machine Age: Work, Progress, and Prosperity in a Time of Brilliant Technologies* (New York: W. W. Norton, 2014).

28. See for instance Robert G. Hollands, "Will the Real Smart City Please Stand Up?," *City* 12, no. 3 (2008): 303–20, doi: 10.1080/13604810802479126; Adam Greenfield, *Against the Smart City* (New York: Amazon Digital Services, 2013); Anthony M. Townsend, *Smart Cities: Big Data, Civic Hackers, and the Quest for a New Utopia* (New York: W. W. Norton, 2014).

29. Hal R. Varian, "Innovation, Components and Complements," 2003, accessed January 18, 2011, at http://www.almaden.ibm.com/coevolution/pdf/varian_paper.pdf.

30. Townsend, *Smart Cities*, 9.

31. For a overview of eight digital master plans, see Anthony Townsend and Stephen Lorimer, "Digital Master Planning: An Emerging Practice in Global Cities,"

NYU Marron Institute of Urban Management Working Paper No. 25, New York, 2015, accessed August 14, 2015, at http://marroninstitute.nyu.edu/uploads/content/Working_Paper_25_Digital_Master_Planning.pdf.

32. Anthony Townsend, *Making Sense of the New Urban Science*, New York University Wagner School, Rudin Center for Transportation Policy and Management, July 2015, accessed September 10, 2015, at www.citiesofdata.org/making-sense-of-the-science-of-cities/.

33. Kevin Bullis, "Smart Forecasts Lower the Power of Wind and Solar," *MIT Technology Review*, April 23, 2014, accessed September 2, 2015, at www.technologyreview.com/featuredstory/526541/smart-wind-and-solar-power/.

34. For further background on human task routing, see "The Future of Coordination: A Toolkit for Making the Future," Institute for the Future, accessed September 2, 2015, at www.iftf.org/coordination/.

35. Townsend, *Smart Cities*, 26.

36. Tim Schröder, "Automation's Ground Floor Opportunity," *Pictures of the Future*, spring 2011, 19, accessed June 5, 2015, at www.siemens.com/innovation/apps/pof_microsite/_pof-spring-2011/_pdf/pof_0111_strom_buildings_en.pdf.

37. Eric Paulos and James Pierce, "Citizen Energy: Towards Populist Interactive Micro-Energy Production," Hawaii International Conference on System Science (HICSS) Kauai, 2011.

38. Townsend, *Making Sense of the New Urban Science*.

39. Anthony Townsend and Alissa Chisholm, *Citizen Urban Science: New Partnerships for Advancing Knowledge*, Cities of Data Project, New York University Wagner School, Rudin Center for Transportation Policy and Management, August 2015, accessed September 2, 2015, at www.citiesofdata.org/report-citizen-urban-science/.

40. R. Jordan, A. Crall, S. Gray, T. Phillips, and D. Mellor, "Citizen Science as a Distinct Field of Inquiry," *BioScience* (2015), doi: 10.1093/biosci/biu217.

41. "Teaching with Documents: Court Documents Related to Martin Luther King, Jr., and Memphis Sanitation Workers," National Archives, accessed July 25, 2015, at www.archives.gov/education/lessons/memphis-v-mlk/.

42. U.S. Environmental Protection Agency, "Summary of Executive Order 12898—Federal Actions to Address Environmental Justice in Minority Populations and Low-Income Populations," overviews and factsheets, accessed July 26, 2015, at www2.epa.gov/laws-regulations/summary-executive-order-12898-federal-actions-address-environmental-justice.

43. Robert D. Bullard and Glenn S. Johnson, "Environmentalism and Public Policy: Environmental Justice: Grassroots Activism and Its Impact on Public Policy Decision Making," *Journal of Social Issues* 56, no. 3 (2000): 555–78, doi:10.1111/0022-4537.00184.

44. Jason Corburn, "Environmental Justice, Local Knowledge, and Risk: The Discourse of a Community-Based Cumulative Exposure Assessment," *Environmental Management* 29, no. 4 (2002): 451–66.

45. Cathy C. Conrad and Krista G. Hilchey, "A Review of Citizen Science and Community-Based Environmental Monitoring: Issues and Opportunities," *Environmental Monitoring and Assessment* 176, nos. 1–4 (2011): 273–91, doi:10.1007/s10661-010-1582-5.

46. Townsend and Chisholm, "Citizen Urban Science."

47. Nick Sinai and Gayle Smith, "The United States Releases Its Second Open Government National Action Plan," White House, December 6, 2013, accessed August 5, 2015, at www.whitehouse.gov/blog/2013/12/06/united-states-releases-its-second-open-government-national-action-plan.

48. Jennifer Pahlka quoted in Townsend, *Smart Cities*, 291.

49. Tom Kalil at VIP Keynote Plenary Session, Global City Teams Challenge Expo, June 1, 2015, Washington, D.C.

50. "World Urbanization Prospects: The 2007 Revision"; Blake Alcott, "Jevons' Paradox," *Ecological Economics* 45, no. 1 (2005): 9–21.

# It Is Easier to Be Smart
# than to Be Green

DISCUSSANT: MOIRA ZELLNER
UNIVERSITY OF ILLINOIS AT CHICAGO

Our panel focused on the notion of the smart city and its potential to address difficult environmental issues through the use of various forms of digital technology, among them sensed, simulated, and communicated data; computational models, operations and management algorithms; and data mining techniques. Although human ingenuity has given rise to an incredible number of digital tools that are cheaper to access and use, this does not automatically translate into social and environmental improvements. Moreover, despite the advances in the areas of data science, big data, urban informatics, and urban analytics, humanity as a whole is still struggling to figure out how to shift gears and operationalize concepts such as sustainability and resilience. This is a much larger issue than the question of how to use our tools. It's about what we might want to use our tools for.

To start this conversation, we might want to distinguish among the following:

1. Data: facts or measurements collected for further analysis (note: further analysis should be the purpose of collecting data)

2. Information: what is conveyed or represented by the analysis of data
3. Knowledge: the implications for action derived from the information
4. Wisdom: the lessons learned over time, as we evaluate the impacts of our actions relative to our expectations and values.[1]

It's important not to confuse data with information. A datum means very little unless contrasted with another datum to derive meaning, even if implicitly. This meaning is information. A single temperature value by itself means little. Even a time series of data means little, unless we look at each datum relative to each other, or relative to a different time series. I infer that it is cold or hot today because I implicitly compare the value I read in the thermometer with my own body temperature. Without some form of analysis, data mean little.

Without applying analysis to action, there is little use for information. Knowledge is sometimes, too, confused with information. Rather, knowledge is derived from putting information to practical use. This "so what?" question is critical if our goal is to change. Finally, without the capacity to learn from these experiences, knowledge cannot grow. And without wisdom, there is little chance of adaptation, transformation, and survival.

There is no single or best way to be smart, and gathering and manipulating data alone does not make us more knowledgeable or wise. Current efforts tend to overemphasize data collection and pattern identification, paying less attention to its meaning for action or to examining unintended consequences of technology. The use of data and information to create knowledge and wisdom is a social issue, part of the social contract that this Urban Forum focuses on. It is as much—or more—about humans as it is about the technology that we develop to create smart cities.

Technology by itself is neither a solution nor a guarantee for improvement unless humans use it to solve our persistent complex social and environmental problems. Our society tends to fetishize technology to the point of forgetting the problem that it is supposed to address.[2] The danger in this fascination is that technology is an extremely powerful influence that shapes the way we live, use resources, and relate to one another. Technology can be an incredible ally in providing cures to medical conditions, for example, but it can also be the source of the pollution that causes disease. It can enable us to access an incredible source of energy to power our life, or to destroy it. Technology allowed us to build transportation and construction machines and to support the rise of cities and other socio-infrastructural systems that are hubs of innovation, creativity, and efficiency that feed further inventions, but it has also created demands for resources that were not previously sought after, and in so doing it is dangerously disconnected from the reality of a limited and disparate world. Technology opens up alternative paths; our choice of path will set processes in motion that reinforce it, making it difficult to return or change, even as we see red flags. As much as technology is not the solution, it is not the problem, either. The problem and the solution lie in how humans create and use technology, and for what purpose.

Cars were invented to help people travel from one place to another in a city. We ended up building cities *for* cars, setting us into a rigid pattern of excess driving and carbon emissions, storm-water runoff and flooding, among others, from which it is difficult to break away. Building cities managed by information technology can give us a false sense of order and efficiency (being "smart"), but in the combination with human decision making is where things can go awry (being unwise). Examples are a traffic jam of smart Teslas, and the possibility that, not finding a parking space, people would set their autonomous vehicles to drive around while they shop. These are just examples we can think of; there are many possibilities we cannot yet imagine.

Technology has fed our penchant for unlimited growth, which is a biophysical impossibility. We often hear about the benefits of technology in creating opportunities for efficiency gains to accommodate further growth. These gains are only temporary or short-term, for two reasons:

- Whenever gains in efficiency are attained, there is a rebound effect, also known as the Jevons paradox. Many studies show empirical evidence of how, when people save by gains in efficiency, the gains are limited in time. Gradually, people tend to use the savings to consume more of either that same resource or other resources, with the consequent problems of pollution and depletion.
- We cannot reduce our consumption of energy or resources to 0 units per capita—that is, we cannot grow indefinitely. Efficiency gains plateau, as well. We might find substitutes, which delay the plateauing, but resources are limited, either in their absolute values, or in the rates at which they are regenerated. This is more so if human activity has deteriorated environmental resources to the point of diminishing environmental regeneration and treatment capabilities. Many impacts of excessive consumption are delayed or hard to detect because of system feedbacks, but they are real and already happening. Although widely criticized, the model of limits to growth posed by the Meadowses and colleagues has been validated with data over thirty years that suggest humanity is on the business-as-usual track on its way to collapse.[3] Recent studies confirm how drastically marine life has

declined, and the more recent financial and health-care crises are confirmation of this looming contraction.[4]

The fascination with data and technology might give the illusion that we can overcome these limits, and it can prevent us from making adjustments in a timely manner before adjustments are made for us, traumatically. The gains in efficiency that technology can bring are quickly lost without disincentivizing consumption or addressing disparities. We live in a consumerist society, however, which makes this approach politically challenging. Coming up with an attractive way to show how development can happen without increased consumption might give us a way out. So-called smart technologies can contribute with the meaningful visualization of data to help communities create alternative visions of their future, backed by scientific and social knowledge necessary to support wise choices. Paradoxically, those who are excluded from the technological resources we have grown used to and that we have come to depend on (as evidenced whenever we are paralyzed by a failed software system) might be more inventive and flexible to propose and embrace radically new ways of living. And yet, reputation and status play significant roles in where funding and resources are directed for technological advancement, stifling true and inclusionary innovation. This will be an important point to be aware of as we make decisions on how we want to be "smart," or rather (and hopefully), wise.

## Notes

1. Paola Zellner-Bassett (Virginia Polytechnic Institute and State University), personal communication, 2015.

2. S. Mattern, "Methodolatry and the Art of Measure: The New Wave of Urban Data Science," *Places* (November 2013), accessed March 28, 2016, at https://places journal.org.

3. Donella H. Meadows, Dennis L. Meadows, and William W. Behrens III, *The Limits to Growth: A Report for the Club of Rome's Project on the Predicament of Mankind* (New York: Universe Books, 1972); Donella H. Meadows, Dennis L. Meadows, and Jørgen Randers, *Beyond the Limits: Confronting Global Collapse, Envisioning a Sustainable Future* (Post Mills, Vt.: Chelsea Green Publishing, 1992); Donella H. Meadows, Jørgen Randers, and Dennis L. Meadows, *Limits to Growth: The 30-Year Update* (White River Junction, Vt.: Chelsea Green Publishing, 2004); G. Turner, "A Comparison of the Limits to Growth with 30 Years of Reality," *Global Environmental Change* 18 (2008): 397–411.

4. G. Turner, "On the Cusp of Global Collapse? Updated Comparison of the Limits to Growth with Historical Data," *GAIA* 21, no. 2 (2012): 116—24, accessed March 28, 2016, at www.oekom.de/gaia.

# Social Contract Theory and the Public's Health

## A Vital Challenge Past and Present

WILLIAM C. KLING

*UNIVERSITY OF ILLINOIS AT CHICAGO*

EMILY STIEHL

*UNIVERSITY OF ILLINOIS AT CHICAGO*

> A government of the people, by the people, for the people shall not perish from the earth.
>
> —Abraham Lincoln, Gettysburg Address (1863)

Social contract theory describes trade-offs people face between freely pursuing their own self-interests and becoming members of a society.[1] Granting authority to a civil society through its government should provide for systematic and consistent enforcement of societal norms, which in turn should provide benefits to individuals. As such, individual members of society can experience greater cooperation with others in that society and protection from random acts of individuals. At the same time, citizens forfeit some of their own unregulated freedoms as they grant legitimacy to the socially constructed entities designed to protect them.[2] In the United States, social contract theory has been used to justify programs to protect and advance the health, safety, and welfare of its citizens.[3] For instance, limits on smoking by individuals were developed to protect other members of society from health related risks of second-hand smoke. Individuals socially construct the entities that create these rules and then imbue them with the power to legitimately enforce the rules. One example is the Declaration of Independence, which promises its citizens "Life, Liberty, and the Pursuit of Happiness."[4] This edict serves as the cornerstone of the American public health system.

The development of a society can also accentuate inequality among its members.[5] For instance, individuals who were once freely independent become reliant on and are now compared against other societal members. One potential role of government, then, could be to reduce inequity among the population, and to protect those who are less advantaged. In the United States, the government has become responsible for developing a vast and complex regulatory system to meet, among other things, basic human needs related to food, water, shelter, and heat. Various governmental laws and regulations have established institutions in which to house or assist ill, disabled, and dying populations; developed vaccines and other medicines to prevent the spread of communicable disease; placed restrictions on dangerous and risky behavior; dedicated significant and public resources to research; and developed interventions for mitigating chronic diseases. Federal, state, and local governments, as the conduits for society, have enacted public health laws and regulations implemented through public health departments, public hospitals and clinics, and other institutions.[6]

Most recently, social contract theory has been invoked to justify a social commitment to the provision of individualized health care services. Under this social contract, citizens surrender their ability to opt out of insurance coverage in exchange for improved access to care. Health care costs are distributed across the population in order to accomplish two goals: individuals cannot be denied service when their health care needs become very costly, and health insurance coverage is expanded to previously uninsured individuals.[7] In addition, governmental initiatives have served to develop and support the health care workforce, training a range of health care professionals, including physicians, nurses, physician assistants, and medical technicians, as well as more contemporary jobs such as community health workers and patient navigators. These occupations are integral to the government's objective to protect the health and safety of a sizable and growing aging population.[8] In fact, according to the U.S. Department of Labor, Bureau of Labor Statistics, occupations and industries related to health care are projected to add the most new jobs of any sector between 2012 and 2022, totaling 5 million of the 15.6 million new jobs.[9]

Finally, it is worth noting that public and private workplaces are increasingly being implicated as key players in civil society's protection of its individuals. About half of U.S. residents (53.9%) are covered by employer-sponsored health insurance.[10] And employer contributions seem to have an impact on employee behaviors, influencing the degree to which sick employees continue to work (even when sick or injured) to maintain their employer-sponsored health insurance coverage.[11] This alone raises interesting issues involving social contract theory, since these organizations are not necessarily legitimated by society to provide for the well-being of its citizens. Also confusing is the role of these entities compared to citizens. Private corporations now have the same rights as individual citizens, despite the fact that they typically control far more resources. Yet, employees spend a large portion of their time in the workplace, making it an intriguing partner or context for addressing the health needs of the population. For instance, the workplace could be a site for implementing governmental interventions designed to enhance worker wellness. Employers could contribute to the social contract by investing in training around healthy eating or designing the job to enhance opportunities for exercise.

The role of the social contract among social entities, like employers and individuals, for improving society's health and wellness is even more challenging in the health care industry, where organizations are responsible for protecting the wellness of citizens in their communities, as well as of their employees. Their workers (e.g., nurses, community health workers, allied professionals) provide health care to the larger population but the quality of care they are able to provide is dependent on their own well-being.[12] This juxtaposition of the role of individuals in the workplace versus their role as caregivers in society sets up a complex tension, exacerbated by variables such as income and geography. Health care employers are challenged by their conflicting responsibilities between proving high quality—but not too costly—care to the community, and providing living wages and manageable work arrangements for their employees. As a result, the private and public workplace is an integral and important component of the larger civil society influencing health both for its employees and the community at large.

This paper briefly discusses social contract theory and outlines the state of public health and public health care within that framework. It describes how the workplace in general and the health care workplace in particular serve as societal drivers for the provision of health and health care. It then applies social contract theories to societal expectations related to the police power, citing innovative examples of how the government can better meet its obligations under its public health-related social contract.

## THE COMMON GOOD: SOCIAL CONTRACT THEORIES

Traditional and contemporary social contract theories provide a lens by which to evaluate how our society meets the basic needs of its people. The bedrock concept of the common good and civil society's obligations to protect it has been legitimized through the philosophical works of Thomas Hobbes, John Locke, Jean-Jacques Rousseau, and John Rawls, among others. Under social contract theory, individuals forfeit certain personal freedoms to grant social entities, including governments, the authority to provide for a common good. This could include opportunities for better coordination, cooperation, or efficiency among citizens, by protecting against arbitrary acts from random, unconnected individuals; or opportunities to enhance equity among citizens and reduce asymmetries, by emphasizing social welfare and placing constraints on powerful leaders.[13]

Contemporary social contract theory scaffolds traditional theory by parsing out motives and objectives of individuals vis-à-vis governments. Thus, subjectivists look to each person's individual interests as a justification for political action. For instance, David Gauthier uses the example of the two farmers whose fields will be ready for harvesting at different times.[14] According to modern interpretations of social contract theory, the second farmer may be hesitant to help the first farmer harvest her crop, out of concern that the first farmer will not reciprocate this action when the second farmer is ready to harvest at a later point in time. The first farmer would be in an advantageous position and would be personally better off, at that moment, not helping the other farmer to harvest his crop, thus keeping supply lower.[15] In the same way, even though limiting hazardous plant emissions might be beneficial for society, it is costly for individual organizations to invest resources to control emissions. For this reason, governments are granted power by their citizens to regulate actions that promote the well-being of society as a whole while potentially inconveniencing certain individuals. So, the government may incentivize farmers to jointly increase productivity, or it may limit or control hazardous plant emissions. Two other modern social contract theories examine how citizens consider the needs of others. First, Rawlsian theory looks to the common, shared interests of individuals to justify political action.[16] Here, it is the joint interests of citizens in the larger society that ignite action. For instance, the citizens' need for health care access, and health care entities' increasing costs, drove governments' health care intervention. Second, another theory presents the idea that individuals in society might willingly relinquish their own benefits for the good of others.[17] For example, some individuals would pay income taxes to fund entitlement programs that improve the conditions for those less well off. These modern theorists seem to define the exercise of the authority based on a collective of individuals in a preexisting and changing environment.[18]

Social contract theory does not itself represent a formal contract among a society and its citizens, nor does it formally grant power to a governmental entity. Instead, it is a socially constructed understanding between the citizens—who willingly forgo certain rights in order to reap the benefits of a civil society—and that society. However, in regulating and enforcing the informal contract between a group of citizens and their society, governments do tend to enact laws and develop contracts to formalize the rights and responsibilities of members. Next we highlight some of the laws and contracts that have been developed to reinforce the norms and expectations underlying an efficient society.

## THE LEGAL CONTEXT

In the eyes of the law, "a contract is a promise or a set of promises for the breach of which the law gives a remedy, or the performance of which the law in some way recognizes as a duty." Further, "the formation of a contract requires a bargain in which there is a manifestation of mutual assent to the exchange and a consideration."[19] The social contract is not legally binding; instead, it represents the perceptions of its citizens. However, without some formal understanding, it can be difficult for citizens to fully understand their rights and responsibilities and those of society, including the responsibility of the government to protect its people, as well as the people's responsibility to comply with governmental rules for implementing such protections. Accordingly, "a major part of the agreement is that citizens give up their position as the ultimate law, reposing that power in a representative government that is itself subject to law."[20]

Another way that governments can enforce the rights and responsibilities of their citizens is through the concept of police power, which traditionally has been used to justify the government's legislative authority to "promote public health, public safety, and public morality."[21] Notably, the police powers are conferred through the U.S. Constitution and its sister state constitutions, which set forth the rules by which government governs. If the government acts beyond its constitutional limits of protecting the public health, safety, and welfare, the government's actions may be found unconstitutional and, therefore, unenforceable.[22] Thus, for instance, when the government goes beyond its authority to protect its citizens by unlawful detainment, "stop and frisk," repression of speech, taking of property, or denial of due process, the citizens can formally confront the violation of their social contract.[23]

Throughout our constitutional history, the extent of governmental policy has changed depending on the given political and social climate and context.[24]

Thus, as it relates to the First Amendment, for instance, the court's decisions have consistently reflected "Lockean liberal individualism" during peaceful times, and "Machiavellian civic republicanism" during times of conflict.[25] This changing environment is often analogized to a swinging pendulum, swinging between individual rights and government intervention.[26] For instance, while the government through its police power may require a child to provide proof of immunizations before attending school, an exception is carved out in some jurisdictions for those with religious or moral objection to such immunizations. Indeed, the U.S. Centers for Disease Control and Prevention (CDC) has a two-page document directed at parents who choose not to vaccinate their children.[27]

Arguably, parents so choosing are potentially breaching the social contract, despite the existence of regulations policing these behaviors. Without widespread immunization, diseases that are virtually eradicated or at the least highly manageable place people, particularly children, at risk. The dire nature of this conundrum is illustrated by the Vermont commissioner of public health's plea for people to rethink the importance of vaccinations. Shortly after the 2014 Disneyland measles outbreak, the commissioner called for people to vaccinate their children. In the document he cited that a "dangerous situation" resulted because

> most of the current patients [in the Disneyland outbreak] are unvaccinated. Yes, this outbreak is a result of parents choosing not to vaccinate their children.
>
> There is no controversy. Giving vaccines, like the MMR vaccine that protects against measles, mumps and rubella, is the most important action parents can take to protect their children from illness or death. . . .
>
> Given our society's value of individual rights, it is important to understand that with those rights come responsibilities. Vaccinating our children is part of the social contract."[28]

Another example relates to the Ebola outbreak in 2015. During the crisis, the CDC issued health travel warnings and the U.S. State Department required passengers traveling from virus-originating countries to enter the United States through one of five airports with "enhanced entry screening."[29] This unprecedented quarantine restriction demonstrates how quickly the pendulum can swing. Generally, in order for a quarantine to be valid, it must be a proportionate and appropriate response to the threat. It also must be designed to present the "least infringement" possible. For the public to respond in a positive manner and to uphold its duty to comply with this part of the social contract, the governmental response must be appropriate.[30] If not, the people could perceive the government to have breached the social contract.

Thus, social contract theory provides a framework for assessing the relationship between governmental policies and societal well-being, including the public health and health care needs of its people. The government exercises its duty to protect its people from health-related threats. At the same time, the government's exercise of its authority must be reasonable and rational, and within the confines of constitutionality. Individuals must also act responsibly, both as discrete members of the society and within the context of the greater community. Ultimately, both parties to this "contract"—the government and the people—must act responsibly and with an eye toward their respective duties.

## PUBLIC HEALTH

Government has regulated factors influencing basic human survival for centuries. For instance, the discipline of public health is often said to have originated when John Snow, a well-respected epidemiologist, linked a cholera outbreak in London to a single source of polluted water.[31] And, since the inception of the U.S. government, the political and legal system has been fixated on the responsibility to protect citizens from health-related injury, the spread of disease, and death. For example, laws relating to quarantine, vaccine, and controlling contagion go as far back as the original colonists.[32]

In "celebrating a century of success," the CDC enumerates the "Ten Great Public Health Achievements in the 20th Century" in the United States as follows: immunizations; motor-vehicle safety; workplace safety; control of infectious diseases; decline in deaths from heart disease and stroke; safer and healthier foods; healthier mothers and babies; family planning; fluoridation of drinking water; and recognition of tobacco as a health hazard.[33] One wonders, then, why our society appears to be lagging in so many of these areas. If the social contract is designed to promote the greater good, why are our infant mortality rates, teen pregnancy rates, tobacco usage, accident rates, and so on still so high, particularly as compared to other Westernized countries? Our current infant mortality rate is around 6 in 1,000 births, and the rate among some aspects of the country, especially rural areas with large minority populations, is even higher. In some cases, the rates in these areas more closely resemble rates in developing countries than in the United States. Other Western countries are much lower.[34] Similarly, the teenage live birth rate is 26.5 per 1,000 in the population, making it the highest among

Westernized countries.[35] And, according to the CDC, 18 in 100 (or 42 million) adults still smoke tobacco, accounting for 480,000 deaths each year.[36] These summary data demonstrate that, at least in these three key indicator areas, our public health system does not appear to be meeting its obligations to protect its citizens or reduce inequity under the social contract.

Yet, our government couches the discussion with the assumption that progress has been made since "public health [in these areas] is credited with adding 25 years to the life expectancy of people living in the United States in [the 20th] Century."[37] While admirable and indeed a demonstration of great progress, unhealthy outcomes like infant mortality, teenage pregnancy, and smoking are rampant, and in many sectors of our society, continuing to grow. More urgently, many of these factors are higher in disparate communities, making health disparities a high societal priority. The National Institutes of Minority Health and Health Disparities "envisions an America in which all populations will have an equal opportunity to live long, healthy and productive lives."[38]

In 2010, the U.S. Department of Health and Human Services announced its Healthy People 2020 Initiative, the goals of which are to "attain high-quality, longer lives free of preventable disease, disability, injury, and premature death; achieve health equity, eliminate disparities, and improve the health of all groups; create social and physical environments that promote good health for all; and promote quality of life, healthy development, and healthy behaviors across all life stages."[39] Embedded in the Website are detailed data sets, which upon cursory exploration again seem to belie the underlying notion that our public health social contract is working. According to the Healthy People 2020 Leading Health Indicators Program Update in March 2014, four indicators have met or exceeded targets, ten indicators are improving, eight indicators show little change, and three indicators are worsening.[40] One interesting example that tells an important story is that, while adult cigarette smoking is decreasing (thus categorized as "improving"), adolescent tobacco use is "getting worse."[41] While progress in key public health-related areas gives rise to hope and optimism, "nudging" our government agencies and administrators and people to better recognize and appreciate the balance between the government's promise and duty to protect, and the people's promise and duty to make good choices is essential to a high-functioning society.[42]

To expand on the immunization issue mentioned earlier, while vaccines are identified as one of the top public health priorities in the CDC's Healthy People 2020, our immunization rates are still low, and a growing segment of the population seems inclined to disregard the research and not immunize.

The result? As previously discussed, an outbreak of measles that started at, of all places, Disneyland.[43] Again, where is the systemic breakdown? According to the World Health Organization, immunizations work, deterring up to 3 million deaths per year from diphtheria, tetanus, pertussis, and measles.[44] At the same time, many recommended vaccination rates do not meet the Healthy People 2020 goals.[45] The CDC publishes a fact sheet that explains conditions before immunization programs and warns that we could return to those conditions if we cease vaccinating.[46] In this case, it appears our government is trying desperately to maintain vaccination rates. Yet the public seems confused about its duty to immunize. Maybe it is time for our society to say "enough is enough," as one author puts it.[47]

In addition to these traditional public health indicators, our government has developed a multifaceted and broad-based approach to addressing environmental issues. In terms of the social contract and public trust, the U.S. Supreme Court has established a very low threshold for individuals or groups to have standing to challenge defendants in environmental cases. In order to file a lawsuit, the standing doctrine typically requires plaintiffs to have a personal interest and have suffered some direct injury. In environmental cases, however, individuals and groups have standing to challenge damage to the environment more generally.[48] Thus, under the social contact, individuals and groups can challenge private or governmental decisions that threaten human health and the environment. And, importantly, the Court has ruled that environmental laws "are intended for the protection of the environment, not for the protection of persons deemed responsible for the consequences of having polluted the environment."[49]

Enacted in 1969, the National Environmental Policy Act created the roadmap for subsequent passage of the Clean Water Act, Clean Air Act, and other legislation.[50] Throughout their history, these important laws have provided excellent examples of government regulation of private rights for the betterment of the public good. And, utilizing a system of formal governmental and informal self-controls has proven effective.[51] An example of how controversial these issues can become relates to water resource management. Our country's water resources are dwindling at alarming rates, yet we continue to widely ignore human impact on climate change.[52] With regard to our water system, the scheme of laws, rules, and regulations at the local, regional, state, and federal levels regulating water quality, water resource management, storm water management, recreational use of waterways, riparian rights, and so on has had a tremendous impact.[53] According to the U.S. Environmental Protection Agency, "the Clean Water Act (CWA) establishes the basic structure for regulating discharges of pollutants into the waters of the United States and regulating quality standards for surface waters."[54] Because of achievements under the CWA, once-dead waterways have actually reemerged as "fishable and swimmable."[55] The impact of the Clean Water Act serves as an example of how the social contract has met expectations.[56] Yet, with regard to water resource management, in 2015 California rationed its water for the first time, and other states may not be far behind.[57]

Similarly, great progress has been made on climate change through the Kyoto Protocol and other treaties. However, our Union of Concerned Scientists and many others continue to raise the alarm of how quickly and dramatically our oceans are rising and our land mass is changing. According to the Union of Concerned Scientists, "global warming is already having significant and harmful effects on our communities, our health, and our climate. Sea level rise is accelerating. The number of large wildfires is growing. Dangerous heat waves are becoming more common. Extreme storm events are increasing in many areas. More severe droughts are occurring in others. We must take immediate action to address global warming or these consequences will continue to intensify, grow ever more costly, and increasingly affect the entire planet—including you, your community, and your family."[58]

At the same time, climate change deniers continue their rallying cry that the science is nonsense. According to Greenpeace, at last count the Koch Brothers have spent at least $79,048,951 on groups denying climate change science since 1997.[59] Even high-level policy makers are engaged in this trickery. In May 2015, the *Los Angeles Times* called out the chair of the House Committee on Science, Space, and Technology, Representative Lamar Smith (R-Texas), as one of the "most eminent and influential climate change deniers in Congress."[60] Arguably climate change deniers breach the social contract by condemning overwhelming scientific evidence supporting the concept of humans impacting climate change.

About the people's obligation toward climate change, Lacasse recently found that many Americans do not rate climate change as important compared to other political issues. Thus, "78% of Democrats compared with 53% of Republicans believe that climate change is occurring, and 72% of Democrats worry about climate change compared with only 38% of Republicans."[61] This obvious disconnect between individuals and communities is a stark example of how perceptions impact the social contract. Why don't the majority of people believe our scientists? Clearly, our well-designed system of checks and balances does not appear to be working in the case of climate change, even as our government continues to negotiate laws, polices, and treaties on climate change.[62]

Without question, the public health challenges facing our government and other governments across the globe are tremendous. While we continue to face historical issues like deterring the spread of contagious diseases, the complexity of our new global community requires us to act with great care as we engage in the obligations we are contracted for. In addition, more recent developments relating to the environment and climate change provide us even greater opportunities to negotiate the terms of a new social contract. The next section explores the particular impacts of Patient Protection and Affordable Care Act, which has monumental effects on the public health social contract.

## THE PATIENT PROTECTION AND AFFORDABLE CARE ACT

The Patient Protection and Affordable Care Act (ACA) of 2010 reformed how individuals obtain and how employers provide health care insurance.[63] These significant changes, while giving rise to considerable political unrest, have provided health care insurance to an additional 16 million Americans.[64] This is only the most recent attempt at developing government policy to enforce citizens' rights to health and well-being as part of the social contract. In 1944, President Franklin Delano Roosevelt enumerated a "second bill of rights" that included "a right to adequate medical care and the opportunity to achieve and enjoy good health."[65] Through the 1935 passage of the Social Security Act, Roosevelt created a foundation for the establishment of government-provided health care. And, the Social Security Act Amendments of 1965 established Medicare—"a hospital insurance program for the aged." From Roosevelt's New Deal to Lyndon Johnson's Great Society, a clear path of government-supported health care was established. The progeny of these efforts was the Patient Protection and Affordable Care Act in 2010.

The ACA (P.L 111-148 [2010]) is a monumental piece of legislation. Without a doubt, it has modified the social contract between the government and the people as it relates to access to health care. According to the U.S. Supreme Court in its June 2015 decision, *King v. Burrell*, "the Patient Protection and Affordable Care Act grew out of a long history of failed health insurance reform." In describing the ACA, the court noted that the ACA adopted four key reforms from previous state-wide efforts: guaranteeing coverage and community ratings; requiring individuals to maintain insurance or be penalized; making health insurance more affordable; and creating insurance exchanges. In upholding portions of the ACA in their controversial decision, the court stated that "Congress passed the Affordable Care Act to improve health insurance markets, not to destroy them. If at all possible, we must interpret the Act in a way that is consistent with the former, and avoids the latter."[66]

## ACA IMPACT ON HEALTH CARE ORGANIZATIONS

Through this monumental legislative change, the ACA highlights society's responsibility to address the needs of an aging and unhealthy population and to satisfy its promise to provide health care to U.S. residents. While monumental, the act has also had incremental effects on discrete stakeholders. For instance, one interesting consequence of the ACA relates to how it has changed the way health care organizations operate. In the health care domain, health care organizations are key players in civil society's protection of public health. Health care organizations address the health needs of the communities in which they operate, and they are reimbursed for the care their employees provide. As the reimbursement becomes value based, organizations are having to change their processes to better track patients in the system to help them manage their health.

Health care organizations are also encouraged to increase the health services and outreach they provide to the community, to manage chronic diseases, and to reduce hospital readmissions. In fact, there has been movement away from reimbursements around the treatment of disease and toward the promotion of wellness. Employees in a variety of health care organizations (e.g., hospitals, nursing homes, federally qualified health centers [FQHCs], and home health agencies) provide care to members of the community as part of their jobs. Sometimes this entails direct health care within the organization, but it can also include outreach and education to members of the community. Increasingly, these employees, as agents of the organization, deliver health care in the community—for example, in community clinics or patients' homes—as opposed to in hospitals or other institutional settings. As a result, health care systems have been developing new organizational forms and partnerships to address their social obligations for the public's health.

At the same time, health care organizations consider two primary trade-offs when fulfilling the social contract in their communities. First, health care entities deciding how best to deliver health care must consider the trade-off between their obligations to provide effective health care (to the community) and to allocate their limited resources judiciously (and sustain the organization). Second, they must balance the needs of their patients and those of their employees.

The first trade-off involves the constant tension many health care organizations wrestle with between providing high-quality care to as many people as possible and providing care that is as cost-sensitive and as efficient as possible. Health care spending in the United States is still high compared to that in other developed nations, but overall spending has slowed since about 2010. The adage "no margin, no mission" puts pressure on hospital administrators to ensure that their organizations reduce costs and maintain enough resources to continue to provide services into the future. At the same time, they must consider their responsibility to provide care to all residents in their communities, including those who are uninsured. To facilitate this responsibility, federal and state governments have traditionally provided reimbursements to hospitals that provide uncompensated care, called charity care. However, reimbursements for charity care are not always enough to cover the costs of providing services.

The ACA has expanded insurance coverage to millions of U.S. residents, increasing the demand for health care services and also improving reimbursements for providing services. The ACA includes incentives for health care entities that coordinate care, promote patient health, and can minimize readmission rates from inadequate or improper care. The focus on health care, as opposed to the treatment of disease, has changed organizational structures and processes to better manage patient needs. It has also affected the types of staff that health care systems employ. For instance, to manage their community's health, many organizations have begun to hire front line staff, including care coordinators, navigators, home health aides or even community health workers.[67] These employees work directly with a broad range of patients to help them track and manage the daily aspects of their care, including scheduling appointments and tracking medication. In long-term care facilities, front-line care workers additionally assist their residents with activities of daily living, including eating, bathing, and ambulating, that the residents cannot complete on their own.

In this way, many health care organizations fulfill their social contract to provide health care services to a growing insured population by expanding their front-line workforce. However, this raises issues about the trade-off that occurs within the organization between the needs of the employees and the needs of the patients. The ACA emphasizes high-quality patient care, but the front-line employees providing the bulk of the direct care to patients receive low wages and few direct incentives for doing so. In fact, the feminized nature of the work and the emphasis on direct care may correspond to the lower wages paid to these employees.[68] The work they do is physically and emotionally demanding, and low wages and few resources (e.g., time and income) make it difficult for these employees to cope with the demands of their job. Instead, front-line employees experience conflicts between work and family demands. For instance, low wages can force employees to trade off between healthy behaviors, which may be more costly, and unhealthy ones, which fit into their schedules or budgets. Instead of cooking a healthy meal at home, busy schedules could lead employees to become more dependent on fast food, which tends to have fewer nutritional benefits. While employees are advised to stay home or rest when they are sick or injured, many employees may continue to work in order to maintain their weekly hours or health insurance benefits.[69]

Similarly, although some health care organizations may facilitate health and wellness training in other organizations, their own employees may not have access to such programs. In summary, health care organizations also experience tension between the health needs of the patients in their communities and their social obligation to their employees' well-being. The passage of the ACA has confounded this tension, redefining the terms of the social health care contract.

Focusing employee health serves a practical purpose to society beyond simply fulfilling the social contract. First, replacing employees in health care is costly, since open positions require new applicants to be recruited, selected, and socialized into the organization. Turnover and absence reduce the consistency of care available to patients and can increase opportunities for accidents or injury or both. In health care especially, patients and employees develop relationships that can improve the delivery of care, as the employees learn about the patients and understand how best to treat the patients' concerns and illnesses. The quality of the human resources practices for employees in the organization can affect the quality of care available to members of the community.[70] Since the employees are responsible for providing direct care to patients, factors that inhibit the employees from doing a good job can result in poorer care for patients. Front-line employees who do not receive basic support from their organizations, including wages and benefits, must find other ways of supporting themselves. For instance, having to work multiple jobs or shifts to earn more money leaves less time for them to spend on family or on community caregiving responsibilities, including looking after children or volunteering in the community.[71] These extra responsibilities can also erode their ability to provide high-quality care to patients in their health care organizations. For instance, Rogers and colleagues[72] found that nurses who worked shifts longer than twelve hours, worked overtime, or worked more than forty hours a week had a significantly higher risk of making an error. Working multiple jobs can lead to fatigue or exhaustion at work, increasing the risk of injury.

## THE WORKPLACE

In addition to describing the responsibilities of individuals (at a micro level) and public health institutions (at a macro level) in a society, social contract theory has also been used to describe the social obligations of workplaces to their constituents, namely communities, individuals, and employees. Workplaces derive value from investing in their communities. For instance, research on corporate social responsibility highlights how the provision of service and outreach can improve the workplace's image among its diverse stakeholders.

Generally, workplaces are expanding their roles as potential targets for healthy interventions for employees. They can provide positive benefits to employees (e.g., money, pride, positive self-image). Since most employees spend a large portion of their time in their places of work, the workplace could be an ideal avenue for intervening to improve their health and well-being. In many cases, it involves employee benefits to health. For instance, employers could give their workers additional resources to improve their health (e.g., time to use organizational fitness amenities, incentives for reducing harmful behaviors, and information to help employees to make healthier decisions).

A separate line of research has examined the employer's responsibility for ensuring that the workplace is a safe environment for employees. Safety climate is a construct that measures employee perceptions of safety in their organizations.[73] It has been associated with safer behaviors in the workplace.[74] Organizations could make an effort to increase the importance of safety in their organizations. The primary drivers of safety climate tend to be perceptions that supervisors value safety and that safety is important to the employees' jobs.[75] Finally, organizations could invest in better or more employee training around safety and health. Organizations could become important sites for developing, testing, and implementing interventions for increasing health promotion activities and improving safety in the workplace. The result could include partnerships between private and public workplaces as a part of the larger civil society influencing health both for its employees and the community at large.

We do not suggest that workplaces are necessarily motivated to improve or responsible for addressing the health needs of citizens in society. In fact, many of the organizational improvements in safety and work design came about through the work of unions and other social groups. However, the point is that one area for advancing a focus on health and well-being as part of the social contract might be a partnership with workplaces or enhanced regulations for ensuring that employers are protecting their workers' health.

## LOOKING TO THE FUTURE

Understanding social contract theory is critical as we consider how civil society should protect the public's health, both individually and as a population. Further, a systems theory approach can be used to integrate the broader theoretical underpinnings as applied to the health care system, health behavior, as well as communicable and chronic disease prevention and intervention. Understanding how individuals and organizations are interconnected becomes a key evaluative inquiry.[76] Using contemporary models such as "governability" can promote efficient and effective utilization of scarce government resources.[77] Thus, evaluating process and outcomes of health interventions can provide additional measurements to determine how our governmental systems are meeting the benefit of the bargain under the social contract.

Further, when we are exploring the application of the social contract to the public's health and health care, it is appropriate to focus on public values. These values "help galvanize citizen allegiance, especially in a democracy."[78] Public health is considered a particular policy domain.[79] Clearly, the government's protection of the public health and the provision of health care are a long-term public value. The concept that government will protect its people is at the core of social contract theory and is static in nature.[80]

At the same time, it is worth considering the role of various entities in contributing to the health and well-being of members of our society. Individuals give up unlimited freedoms to maintain a safe, ordered society. In return, they empower government to provide for the health, safety, and well-being of societal members. Similarly, employers give up unlimited profit to obtain protection and support from the government to advance their missions. Health care organizations, in particular, benefit from federal reimbursements designed to enable them to provide care to all citizens, including those who are uninsured. At the same time, they have responsibilities to their communities to provide that care and to provide a safe workplace for their employees.

Looking forward, the ACA raises important questions about the role of employers in contributing to the social contract around advancing society's health and wellness. Are employers potential partners for increasing the health and wellness of employed populations? The majority of U.S. residents are insured through their employers. Providing health and wellness programs to employees in organizations makes it easier to recruit and target individuals for wellness programs. However, do organizational leaders perceive that they are partners in upholding the social contract and in improving the health and wellness of their employees? Or are they incentivized by other considerations?

What is the future of social contract theory as it relates to public health and health care, and what policy recommendations may serve as a catalyst for conversation? What are the implications of the changing health care and public health environment based on monumental policy changes such as the Affordable Care Act? Is there a new expectation of health care as a right to citizens rather than a privilege? Is there a higher burden for providing services—health care systems, health care professionals, or employers who pay higher rates for their employees' insurance? What are the impacts of the changing environment on individual responsibility? These questions highlight the significance of using social contract theory as a lens to understanding the role of civil society to protect the health and safety of its population.

## CONCLUSION

Protecting the public's health and providing health care to the public are two key functions of our U.S. political system. Historically, our governmental structures at the local, state, and federal levels have developed an infrastructure to address the public health needs of our society. At the same time, over the past century, our government has been building the foundation of a complex health care system to provide necessary and sufficient health care services to its people. And our private sector, through the workplace, provides an extra layer of infrastructure through which to improve individual health and meet employees' health care needs. The obligations and duties of the government, its citizens, and the private sector can be analyzed using contract theory. Thus, all parties promise to perform certain actions that benefit the others. Government promises to enact laws to protect the health, safety, and welfare of its people. The people promise to abide by the laws passed. And the private sector promises to act to provide for its workers. As such, this complex system provides an excellent example of applied social contract theory. Whether the contract is traditional or contemporary, understanding how government interacts with its communities offers insight into how well our government is serving the health and health care needs of its citizens, and what people can do to be more healthy. As a society, we can all gain from the benefit of the bargain as it relates to the public's health and health care.

## Notes

The authors express their appreciation to Professor Alba Alexander for her review and suggestions on previous drafts.

1. T. Hobbes, *Leviathan*, critical edition by Noel Malcolm, Clarendon Edition (Oxford: Oxford University Press, 2012). First published in 1651.

2. A. L. Allen, "Social Contract Theory in American Case Law," *Florida Law Review* 51, no. 1 (1999).

3. *Barnes v. Glen Theatre*, 501 US 560, 1991; S. Legarre, "The Historical Background of the Police Power," *University of Pennsylvania Journal of Constitutional Law* 9, no. 745 (2006).

4. Declaration of Independence, 1776; George Anastaplo, "The Constitution at Two Hundred: Explorations," *Texas Tech Law Review* 22 (1991): 967; Steven G. Calabresi, "Vesting Clauses as Power Grants," *Northwestern Univerity Law Review* 88 (1993): 1377.

5. Jean-Jacques Rousseau, *The Social Contract*, trans. M. Cranston (Harmondsworth: Penguin). First published in 1762.

6. J. G. Hodge Jr., "The Role of New Federalism and Public Health Law," *Journal of Law and Health* 12, no. 309 (1997): 6; Lawrence O. Gostin, "A Theory and Definition of Public Health Law," *Public Health Law Power, Duty, Restraint*, revised & expanded second edition (Berkeley: University of California Press/Milbank Memorial Fund, 2008).

7. Patient Protection and Affordable Care Act, P.L. 111-148 (2010).

8. B. Kumar, K. Sharma, and S. Zodpey, "The Nomenclature and Classification of Human Resources for Health: A Review," *Journal of Health Management* 15, no. 2 (2013): 203–26; O'Byrne 2009.

9. "Employment Projections—2012–2022," news release, Bureau of Labor Statistics, U.S. Department of Labor, USDL-13-2393, December 19, 2013.

10. J. C. Smith and C. Medalia, "Health Insurance Coverage in the United States: 2013," *U.S. Census Bureau Current Population Reports* (Washington, D.C.: U.S. Government Printing Office, 2014), 60–250; H. Janicki, "Employment-Based Health Insurance: 2010," *U.S. Census Bureau Household Economic Studies* 70, no. 134 (February 2013).

11. C. J. Bradley, D. Neumark, and S. Barkowski, "Does Employer-Provided Health Insurance Constrain Labor Supply Adjustments to Health Shocks? New Evidence on Women Diagnosed with Breast Cancer," *Journal of Health Economics* 32, no. 5 (2013): 833–49.

12. "Employment Projections—2012–2022."

13. Rousseau, *The Social Contract*.

14. David P. Gauthier, *Morals by Agreement* (Oxford: Oxford University Press, 1986); G. Hill, "Reason and Will in Contemporary Social Contract Theory," *Political Research Quarterly* 48, no. 1 (1995): 101–16.

15. M. Uzan-Milofsky, "Shall We Be Resolute?," *Rationality and Society* 21, no. 3 (2009): 337–57.

16. John Rawls, *A Theory of Justice* (Cambridge, Mass.: Harvard University Press, 1971); Greg Hill, "Reason and Will in Contemporary Social Contract Theory," *Political Research Quarterly* 48.1 (1995): 101–116.

17. Thomas Nagel, "Death," *Noûs* (1970): 73–80; Thomas Scanlon, "Rights, Liberty, and Property," in *Reading Nozick*, ed. Jeffrey Paul (Totowa, N.J.: Rowman and Littlefield, 1981); Hill, "Reason and Will."

18. M. Verschoor, "The Democratic Boundary Problem and Social Contract Theory," *European Journal of Political Theory*, 2015, doi:10.1177/1474885115572922.

19. Restatement of Contracts, sections 1 and 17.

20. John B. Mitchell, "My Father, John Locke, and Assisted Suicide: The Real Constitution Right," *Indiana Health Law Review* 3 (2006): 45.

21. Legarre, "Historical Background of the Police Power," 787, citing *Mugler v. Kansas*, 123 US 623, 661 (1887).

22. Legarre, "Historical Background of the Police Power," 788.

23. *Mapp v. Ohio*, 367 U.S. 643, 660 (1961); V. C. Jackson, "Constitutional Law in an Age of Proportionality," *Yale Law Journal* 124 (2015): 2680–3203; *Chaplinsky v. New Hampshire*, 315 U.S. 568 (1942); *Matthews v. Eldridge*, 424 U.S. 319, (1976); *United States v. Carmack*, 329 U.S. 230, 241–42 (1946).

24. G. Molander, "Machiavellian Jurisprudence: The United States Supreme Court's Doctrinal Approach to Political Speech under the First Amendment," *Touro Law Review* 10 (1993): 593.

25. Ibid., 598.

26. Mark C. Rahdert, "The Toughest Job Interview in the Land," *Temple Political & Civil Rights Law Review* 2 (1993): 293.

27. "If You Choose Not to Vaccinate Your Child, Understand the Risks and Responsibilities," Information for Parents, Centers for Disease Control and Prevention, March 2012, accessed April 12, 2016, at www.cdc.gov/vaccines/hcp/patient-ed/conversations/downloads/not-vacc-risks-bw-office.pdf.

28. Health Commissioner Harry Chen, "Vaccines Work!," op-ed, Vermont Department of Health, February 11, 2015, accessed April 12, 2016, at http://healthvermont.gov/news/2015/021115_vaccines_work_chen_oped.aspx.

29. "Ebola Fact Sheet for Travelers," *U.S. Passports & International Travel*, U.S. Department of State–Bureau of Consular Affairs, undated, accessed April 12, 2016, at http://travel.state.gov/content/passports/english/go/Ebola.html.

30. M. A. Rothstein, "From SARS to Ebola: Legal and Ethical Considerations for Modern Quarantine," *Indiana Health Law Review* 12, no. 1 (2015): 228–280.

31. Gostin, "A Theory and Definition of Public Health Law," 19.

32. Rothstein, "From SARS to Ebola," 230.

33. "Ten Great Public Health Achievements in the 20th Century," About CDC 24-7, Centers for Disease Control and Prevention, last updated April 26, 2013, accessed April 12, 2016, at www.cdc.gov/about/history/tengpha.htm.

34. "Infant Mortality," Reproductive Health, Centers for Disease Control and Prevention, last updated January 12, 2016, accessed April 12, 2016, at www.cdc.gov/reproductivehealth/MaternalInfantHealth/InfantMortality.htm.

35. "Teen Pregnancy in the United States," About Teen Pregnancy, Centers for Disease Control and Prevention, last updated May 19, 2015, accessed April 12, 2016, at www.cdc.gov/teenpregnancy/about/index.htm.

36. "Current Cigarette Smoking among Adults in the United States," Smoking & Tobacco Use, Centers for Disease Control and Prevention, last updated December 8, 2015, accessed April 12, 2016, at www.cdc.gov/tobacco/data_statistics/fact_sheets/adult_data/cig_smoking/index.htm.

37. Centers for Disease Control and Prevention, "Current Cigarette Smoking among Adults in the United States," 2014.

38. "About NIMHD," National Institutes of Minority Health and Health Disparities, www.nimhd.nih.gov/about/visionMission.html.

39. "About Healthy People," Healthy People 2020, www.healthypeople.gov/2020/About-Healthy-People.

40. Ibid.

41. Ibid.

42. Richard Thaler and Cass Sunstein, *Nudge: Improving Decisions about Health, Wealth, and Happiness* (New Haven, Conn.: Yale University Press, 2008); Cass R. Sunstein, "Irreversibility," *Law, Probability, and Risk* 9.3–4 (2010): 227–245.

43. Adam Nagourney and Abby Goodnough, "Measles Cases Linked to Disneyland Rise, and Debate Over Vaccinations Intensifies," *New York Times*, January 21, 2015.

44. "Immunization Surveillance, Assessment and Monitoring," Immunization, Vaccines and Biologicals, World Health Organization, 2014, accessed April 12, 2016, at www.who.int/immunization_monitoringglobalsummary/timeseries/tswucovveragebcg.html; "Global Immunization Data," World Health Organization, July 2015, www.who.int/immunization/monitoring_surveillance/Global_Immunization_Data.pdf?ua=1.

45. N. Bobo, "Increasing Immunization Rates through the Immunization Neighborhood Recognizing School-Located Immunization Programs," *NASN School Nurse* 29.5 (September 2014): 224–28.

46. "What Would Happen If We Stopped Vaccinations?," Vaccines and Immunizations, Centers for Disease Control and Prevention, May 19, 2014, www.cdc.gov/vaccines/vac-gen/whatifstop.htm.

47. D. Ropeik, "Declining Vaccination Rates: Time for Society to say Enough Is Enough," *Contemporary Pediatrics*, 2011, http://contemporarypediatrics.modern medicine.com/contemporary—pediatrics/news/modernmedicine/modern-medicine-now/declining-vaccination-rates?page=full.

48. C. Warshaw and G. E. Wannier, "Business as Usual? Analyzing the Development of Environmental Standing Doctrine since 1976," *Harvard Law and Policy Review* 5, no. 289 (2011): 289–322, citing *Duke Power v. Caroline Environmental Study Group*,

438 U.S. 59 (1978), accessed February 23, 2016, http://harvardlpr.com/wp-content/uploads/2013/05/5.2_4_Warshaw.pdf.

49. *North Shore Gas Company v. Environmental Protection Agency*, 930 F.2d 1239, 1243 (1991); Warshaw and Wannier, "Business as Usual," 310.

50. Phillip Michael Ferester, "Revitalizing the National Environmental Policy Act: Substantive Adaptations from NEPA's Progeny," *Harvard Environmental Law Review* 16 (1992): 207; Langberg 2014.

51. Karen Umemoto and Krisnawati Suryanata, "Technology, Culture, and Environmental Uncertainty Considering Social Contracts in Adaptive Management," *Journal of Planning Education and Research* 25.3 (2006): 264–274; Andy Bennett, "Subcultures or Neo-tribes? Rethinking the Relationship between Youth, Style, and Musical Taste," *Sociology* 33.3 (1999): 599–617.

52. B. C. Parks and J. T. Roberts, "Climate Change, Social Theory and Justice," *Theory, Culture and Society* 27, nos. 2–3 (2010): 134–66.

53. Clean Water Act, 33 U.S.C. §1251 et seq. (1972).

54. "Summary of the Clean Water Act," Laws & Regulations, United States Environmental Protection Agency, last updated October 8, 2015, accessed April 12, 2016, at www2.epa.gov/laws-regulations/summary-clean-water-act.

55. "Troubled Waters," *NOW with Bill Moyers*, PBS, accessed April 12, 2016, at www.pbs.org/now/science/cleanwater.html; T. D. Abel and J. T. Hennessey, "State and Local Opportunities in Environmental Policy: Cleaning Up the Potomac and Anacostia Rivers," *Public Works Management and Policy* 2, no. 2 (1997): 159–70.

56. Abel and Hennessey, "State and Local Opportunities in Environmental Policy"; G. J. MacDonald, "Environment: Evolution of a Concept," *Journal of Environment and Development* 12, no. 2 (2003): 151–76.

57. Executive Order B-29-15, signed by Governor Brown, April 1, 2015, accessed at https://www.gov.ca.gov/docs/4.1.15_Executive_Order.pdf; Adam Nagourney, "California Imposes First Mandatory Water Restrictions to Deal with Drought," *New York Times*, April 1, 2015, www.nytimes.com/2015/04/02/us/california-imposes-first-ever-water-restrictions-to-deal-with-drought.html?_r=0.

58. "Global Warming: Confronting the Realities of Climate Change," Union of Concerned Scientists, www.ucsusa.org/global_warming#.VZrjETvbKAI.

59. "Koch Industries: Secretly Funding the Climate Denial Machine," Greenpeace, no date, www.greenpeace.org/usa/en/campaigns/global-warming-and-energy/polluterwatch/koch-industries/.

60. Michael Hiltzik, "A Congressional Climate Change Denier's Disingenuous Defense," *Los Angeles Times*, May 6, 2015, www.latimes.com/business/hiltzik/la-fi-mh-a-congressional-climate-change-deniers-20150506-column.html#page=1.

61. K. Lacasse, "The Importance of Being Green: The Influence of Green Behaviors on Americans' Political Attitudes Toward Climate Change," *Environment and Behavior*, 2014, 755–56, doi:0013916513520491.

62. "Climate Change," United States Environmental Protection Agency, last updated January 20, 2016, www.epa.gov/climatechange.

63. Patient Protection and Affordable Care Act, P.L. 11-148 (2010).

64. Health Care Blog, White House (President Barack Obama), https://www.whitehouse.gov/healthreform/blog.

65. G. P. Smith and R. P. Gallena, "Re-Negotiating a Theory of Social Contract for Universal Health Care in America or, Securing the Regulatory State?," *Catholic University Law Review* 63, no. 1 (2014): 1–40.

66. *King v. Burwell*, 135 S. Ct. 475, 190 L. Ed. 2d 355 (2014), slip op., 4–5, 2, 21.

67. Bureau of Labor Statistics, U.S. Department of Labor, "Fastest Growing Occupations," *Occupational Outlook Handbook, 2014–2015 Edition*, 2015, accessed July 3, 2015, at www.bls.gov/ooh/mobile/fastest-growing.htm.

68. P. England, M. Budig, and N. Folbre. "Wages of Virtue: The Relative Pay of Care Work," *Social Problems* 49 (2002): 455–73.

69. Bradley, Neumark, and Barkowski, "Does Employer-Provided Health Insurance Constrain Labor Supply Adjustments to Health Shocks?"

70. S. C. Eaton, "Beyond 'Unloving Care': Linking Human Resource Management and Patient Care Quality in Nursing Homes," *International Journal of Human Resource Management* 11, no. 3 (2000): 591–616.

71. S. E. Taylor, R. L. Repetti, and T. E. Seeman, "Health Psychology: What Is an Unhealthy Environment and How Does It Get under the Skin?," *Annual Review of Psychology* 48 (1997): 411–47.

72. A. E. Rogers, W. T. Hwang, L. D. Scott, L. H. Aiken, and D. F. Dinges, "The Working Hours of Hospital Staff Nurses and Patient Safety," *Health Affairs* 23, no. 4 (2004): 202–12.

73. D. Zohar, "Safety Climate in Industrial Organizations: Theoretical and Applied Implications," *Journal of Applied Psychology* 65, no. 1 (1980): 96–102.

74. D. Zohar and G. Luria, "A Multilevel Model of Safety Climate: Cross-Level Relationships between Organization and Group-Level Climates," *Journal of Applied Psychology* 90, no. 4 (2005): 616–628.

75. D. C. Seo, M. R. Torabi, E. H. Blair, and N. T. Ellis, "A Cross-Validation of Safety Climate Scale Using Confirmatory Factor Analytic Approach," *Journal of Safety Research* 35, no. 4 (2004): 427–45.

76. J. Varghese and V. R. Kutty, "Governability Framework for the Evaluation and Implementation of Complex Public Health Functions," *Evaluation Review* 36, no. 4 (2012): 303–19, 306.

77. Jan Kooiman, *Governing as Governance* (London: Sage, 2003).

78. T. Beck Jørgensen, "Public Values, Their Nature, Stability and Change: The Case of Denmark," *Public Administration Quarterly* 30 (2006): 365–398; R. W. Hefner, "On the History and Cross-Cultural Possibility of a Democratic Ideal," in *Democratic Civility: The History and Cross-Cultural Possibility of a Modern Political Ideal*, ed. R. W. Hefner, 3–49 (New Brunswick, NJ: Transaction Publishers, 1998); B. Bozeman and

J. Johnson, "The Political Economy of Public Values: A Case for the Public Sphere and Progressive Opportunity," *American Review of Public Administration* 45, no. 1 (2015): 61–85, 62.

79. Mary Kathleen Feeney and Barry Bozeman. "Public Values and Public Failure: Implications of the 2004–2005 Flu Vaccine Case," *Public Integrity* 9.2 (2007): 175–190; Bozeman and Johnson, "Political Economy of Public Values," 63.

80. J. E. Stiglitz, *The Price of Inequality* (New York: W. W. Norton, 2012); Bozeman and Johnson, "Political Economy of Public Values," 65.

## Other References

Centers for Disease Control and Prevention. "CDC Reports Uneven Declines in Coronary Heart Disease by State and Race/Ethnicity," press release, October 13, 2011.

Cromby, J., and M. E. Willis. "Nudging into Subjectification: Governmentality and Psychometrics." *Critical Social Policy* 34, no. 2 (2014): 241–59.

DeLeire, T., K. Joynt, R. McDonald, and K. Takeaways. "Impact of Insurance Expansion on Hospital Uncompensated Care Costs in 2014." Office of the Assistant Secretary for Planning and Evaluation, U.S. Health and Human Services, September 2014.

Durant, R. F., Y. P. Chun, B. Kim, and S. Lee. "Toward a New Governance Paradigm for Environmental and Natural Resources Management in the 21st Century?" *Administration and Society* 35, no. 6 (2004): 643–82.

Hartman, M., A. B. Martin, D. Lassman, and A. Catlin. "National Health Spending in 2013: Growth Slows, Remains in Step with the Overall Economy." *Health Affairs* 34, no. 1 (2015): 150–60.

Heisler, E. J. "The US Infant Mortality Rate: International Comparisons, Underlying Factors, and Federal Programs." *Congressional Research Service*, 2012, 1–29.

Jenkins, M. "Ethics and Economics in Community Care." *Critical Social Policy* 21, no. 1 (2001): 81–102.

Jennings, C. P. "Medicare, Past, Present, and Future: A Policy Perspective." *Policy, Politics, and Nursing Practice* 3, no. 1 (2002): 57–65.

Jones, C. B. "Revisiting Nurse Turnover Costs: Adjusting for Inflation." *Journal of Nursing Administration* 38 (2008): 11–18. doi:10.1097/01.NNA.0000295636.03216.6f.

La Morte, M. W. "Rights and Responsibilities in the Light of Social Contract Theory." *Educational Administration Quarterly* 13, no. 3 (1977): 31–46.

Piatak, J. S. "Understanding the Implementation of Medicaid and Medicare Social Construction and Historical Context." *Administration and Society*, 2015, doi:10.1177/0095399715581030.

Ropeik, D. "How Society Should Respond to the Risk of Vaccine Rejection." *Human Vaccines and Immunotherapeutics* 9, no. 8 (2013): 1815–18.

Simon, S. A. "Inherent Sovereign Powers: The Influential Yet Curiously Uncontroversial Flip Side of Natural Rights." *Alabama Civil Rights and Civil Liberties Law Review* 4 (2013): 133.

Waldron, J. "It's All for Your Own Good." *New York Review of Books*, October 9, 2014.

Zohar, D. "The Effects of Leadership Dimensions, Safety Climate, and Assigned Priorities on Minor Injuries in Work Groups." *Journal of Organizational Behavior* 23, no. 1 (2002): 75–92.

# Social Contracts and the Problem of Asymmetries

DISCUSSANTS: ALBA ALEXANDER, UNIVERSITY OF ILLINOIS AT CHICAGO
JULIE MORITA, CHICAGO DEPARTMENT OF PUBLIC HEALTH
NORBERT G. RIDELL, NAUREX
TERRY VANDEN L. HOEK, DEPARTMENT EMERGENCY MEDICINE, UIC

What constitutes the social contract in the realm of public health? The panel title defines the poles of the debate: is health care a privilege or a right? President Obama similarly framed the choices when he affirmed, "we believe that access to affordable health care isn't a privilege—it's a right."[1] He criticized the more than twenty states that then resisted expanding their Medicaid programs, therefore reinforcing their stance on health care as a privilege for those with insured employers or able to pay through private means.[2] The U.S. Supreme Court ruled in 2012 that states could opt out of the Patient Protection and Affordable Care Act's (ACA) provision for Medicaid expansion.[3] It is strange to call something a right if a large fraction of the population lacks the means to obtain it. Panel moderator Julie Morita, Chicago Commissioner of Public Health, therefore was noticeably strained in trying to portray the Affordable Care Act as an "evolution" from Medicare and Medicaid.[4] Is the "social contract" out of which Medicare and Medicaid grew the same as the one the ACA purported to fulfill? Morita spoke of "different social contracts" occurring over time, for good reason.

Through expanded Medicaid, the ACA aimed to reduce the long-term uninsured disproportionately centered among low-income earners. Medicaid eligibility criteria in the states before the Affordable Care Act excluded "childless adults" and was limited to adults with children whose median income in 2015 was no more than 44 percent of the federal poverty level (about $8,800 for a family of three). The landmark health care legislation in 2010 increased eligibility to include low-income individuals with incomes at or below 138 percent of the federal poverty level. Yet, in line with President Obama's reference, more than 3 million adults remain uninsured in the states that refused to expand Medicaid coverage.[5] Millions more lie outside such coverage for a host of other reasons.

What do we learn from the panel about how a social contract around public health is defined or, more to the point, being redefined today? The most telling response was spelled out in the paper by William Kling and Emily Stiehl. In the conference version of their paper, they had assumed that a social contact in public health is working according to highly limited criteria. For this book they amend their assessment of a social contract in public health and question its effectiveness according to a few additional indicators. They now take a more critical stance on how effectively a social contract in public health is holding up. So I focus my comments here on the panel's criteria for assessments and on the panelists' wavering definition of social contract.

Panelist coauthors Kling and Stiehl apply social contract theory in order to understand the provision of U.S. health care. The Affordable Care Act they examine is an event with the power to change the character of the average American's existence for good or ill, or both. The means of this change is mandated health care access that is employment-based and privately financed but underwritten by federal subsidies and guarantees. My earlier concern still stands: equating social contract with legal contract, as they do, erodes the critical evaluative power of a social contract framework. The "fix" would have been easy if they acknowledged the distinction and worked from there, but they did not understand the point because they are committed to a conceptual frame of "state versus individuals" with no intervening powerful actors and organizations to be accounted for. Their notion of "right" also only amounts to the formal right that a poor family has to purchase a new Ferrari or the Hope Diamond, if they like. This highly limited yet all-too-familiar market conception of "right" leads to analytical dead ends.

## THE CONCEPT OF THE SOCIAL CONTRACT

Kling and Stiehl, and the majority of the panel, present social contract as a partnership broadly between government and its people, and refer to civil society as executing its moral and ethical obligations to protect the public health. The authors needed to distinguish carefully between social contract theory in political philosophy, in which it is the basis for political legitimacy (where the citizenry, not the judges, are the judge), and contract theory in law, where the courts form the entire universe. There are areas of overlap, but the areas where they do not overlap are vital political concerns. All the panelists slipped into conflating social contract in political theory with contracts in law. Only contract theory in law was left standing, shorn of the critical standards that social contract in political theory can bring to bear on its inherent political and social shortcomings. Terry Vanden Hoek is an exception in that he stuck to emergency room experiences to illustrate on-the-ground effects.

Kling and Stiehl continue to assume that once a social contract occurs—or, more so the case, is reckoned to have occurred—it must have been freely agreed and, furthermore, that it accords with the protective function it should perform. To be fair, in their terms neither single-payer nor the Affordable Care Act meets the needs of the social contract in health care, but once one or the other is selected, however it happens, then in their restrictive view the game is over and the contract is fulfilled. All but one panelist seemed in accord with this analytical tack. Can we not have criteria by which to judge whether one arrangement or the other better suits and meets the public needs? None of the panelists defined what public well-being is or ventured to examine the changing public historical understanding of it.

Critics long ago noticed that asymmetries of power among bargainers are concealed by legal forms. Rousseau agreed that these underlying asymmetries adversely affect the social contract: "Do you want coherence in the state? Then bring the two extremes as close together as possible, have neither very rich men nor beggars, for these two estates, naturally inseparable, are equally fatal to the common good; from the one comes friends of tyranny, from the other, tyrants."[6] The authors omit this crucial factor of differential power among agents because in courts of law it does not matter. Politically, the social contract after Hobbes has come to signify a means by which weaker parties impose constraints—not so much on each other, but on their rulers, to save the "commonwealth" from arbitrary, one-way advantages for elites. In patrimonial relations there supposedly were mutual responsibilities binding lord and peasant, but the reality depended on actual power.[7] So a social contract foremost is a curb on arbitrariness, and because this arbitrariness is usually curbed in degrees, the content of the social contract is never final. All social contract theories from Hobbes to Freud are just-so stories, not empirical explanations, and thus are arguments designed to demonstrate the payoffs of a trade-off of liberty or license for a binding contract securing welfare for all. As Hampton deduced, "there is no literal social contract in any successful social contract theory."[8]

Moreover, twentieth-century reformulations have shaped our understanding of the social contract and went unacknowledged on the panel. Note the touchstone work of R. G. Collingwood, who proposed a "postwar social contract" that in many particulars, especially the National Health Service, came to fruition in Britain.[9] To the classics' emphasis on political consent and popular sovereignty, Collingwood adds commitment to social welfare (a safety net) and the reduction of inequality. Industrial societies after the economic and political crises of the 1930s and 1940s incorporated these aspirations. Many social protections were added, which swelled the ranks of the middle class.[10]

Social contracts can be imposed. Bismarck's Germany is an instructive example where authorities possess ample power and the populace must take what is on offer.[11] Given a consistent majority public opinion in favor of British- or Canadian-style single-payer, the passage of the Affordable Care Act (born of a report from the conservative Heritage Foundation) has many features disturbingly in common with that situation.[12] The trickiest aspect is the attendant assumption that anything declared a social contract necessarily must improve equity. The social actors as abstractions are deemed all equal when the various resources they actually bring to bear determine the outcomes. Hence, they presuppose an outcome of equality versus actually achieving it.[13] Consider that under the U.S. social contract—if we may dub it such—the "life, liberty and pursuit of happiness" of corporations, which are considered "persons" under U.S. Supreme Court rulings, is guaranteed as much and indeed much more (because of their resources) than that of flesh and blood persons. Philosophically, the authors' concept of social contract begins and ends with Hobbes, for whom the imperative was subordination of a feral public of disaggregated individuals to a single dominant authority. Questions of justice and equity do not arise lest they disturb the Leviathan's order, which is all that need concern them about the fine print of the social contract. Legal authorities may be content with this situation, but it will not be the case for most political theorists, philosophers, sociologists, historians, and a host of other actors concerned about the vicissitudes of the social contract at any point in the shifting historical balance of competing interests.

## NATIONAL HEALTH CARE: ON THE RISE OR ON THE ROPES?

The assiduously avoided problem in the panel discussion is that private provision of care is now mandatory and is a guaranteed income boon for private insurance companies, already moving toward tighter oligopoly, which begs the question of who this social contract primarily serves. Only panelist Norbert Riedel mentioned that employer provision of health care cannot possibly be universal or even adequate for the entire population. Kling and Stiehl, for example, laud employers who "invest" in the health of their employees when, to the contrary, we see employers everywhere over decades offloading costs onto employees in constant "givebacks." Health care expenditures are the fastest growing component of employee compensation. As a percentage of wages and salaries, health care costs increased fourfold between 1965 and 1990 alone. In response, U.S. firms reduced coverage. Kling and Stiehl cite a 1991 U.S. Supreme Court decision geared "for the protection of the environment, not for the protection of persons deemed responsible for the consequences of having polluted the environment."[14] They imply that this is how health care will work out under the Affordable Care Act framework. It is easy, though, for critics to mount an argument that the Affordable Care Act protects less of the citizenry's health than the very agents whose private provision of health care was the source of the problem to begin with. The Obama administration dropped the public option. So with whom is the public health social contract actually forged? A wider social contract view can bring a critical eye to the context in which the legal and legislative elements of the contract are devised.

Finally, the lack of historical context still leaves us with troubling misconceptions of the dynamics of "public and private workplaces" as "key players in civil society's protection of its individuals." Kling and Stiehl stated on the panel that "the private sector promises to act maternally and paternally to provide for its workers. As such, this complex system provides an excellent example of applied social contract theory." They maintain this misleading portrayal. The authors write about safety provisions as if safety is the gift of the caring employers, when virtually every workplace safety improvement in the last century came about through worker action and union organizing. The authors need to account for an incessant corporate push since the 1970s for deregulation so that these firms can diminish their legal—let alone ethical—responsibilities to the workforce, local communities, and the state.

Regarding the Affordable Care Act, the insurance industry has not given up "unlimited profit," as Kling and Stiehl claim, and have not even slowed the rate at which they seek it, if one scans the business pages. To say "our private sector, through the workplace, provides an extra layer of infrastructure through which to improve individual health and meet employees' health care needs" remains unconvincing. The "extra layer of infrastructure" among health providers siphons at least 30 percent in administrative costs (versus a fraction of that in public systems).[15]

I asked Kling and Stiehl to consider whether "government intervention" and "individual rights" really exist in zero-sum relation, and all they did was reaffirm this belief without argument or evidence. Government programs can and do boost the bargaining power of individuals (e.g., public health care, unemployment compensation, housing benefits, subsidized education) versus powerful private actors and thereby can raise the overall well-being of the nation.[16] It is difficult, though, to see how a program demanding that the least well-paid full-time employees be compelled to pay private insurance rates for health care is a boon to those workers, especially when demonstrably effective programs like the public option were available.

Where the panelists inject some notion of class and status differences, they need to take them seriously, not just mention them briefly and go on. The rollback of historic commitments negotiated between organized labor and employers in the postwar period is a major element contributing to decreasing security of middle classes. There is no mention of these trends among the central stakeholders of the postwar social contract. Instead, we are told that "the workplace in general and the health care workplace in particular serve as societal drivers for the provision of health and health care." With one welcome exception, the panelists, doubtless out of a misplaced sense of practicality, confined themselves to discussion of the social contract within the terms of the Affordable Care Act, as if it were the perfect consummation of a social contract, when it more likely is just the beginning stage of a longer legislative road to the realization and provision of public health care.

## Notes

1. The White House (President Barack Obama), Office of the Press Secretary, "Remarks by the President at Burke for Governor Rally," October 28, 2014, accessed 22 October 2015 at ww.whitehouse.gov.

2. Jeffrey Young, "In States that Didn't Expand Medicaid, It's as if Obamacare Doesn't Even Exist for the Poor," *Huffington Post*, July 10, 2014, accessed 24 October 2015 at www.huffingtonpost.com; "Status of State Action on the Medicaid Expansion Decision," Henry Kaiser Family Foundation, September 1, 2015, accessed 21 October 2015 at http://kff.org.

3. Adam Liptak, "Supreme Court Upholds Health Care Law, 5–4, in Victory for Obama," *New York Times*, June 28, 2012.

4. In addition to moderator Julie Morita, the panel consisted of William C. Kling, Emily Stiehl, Norbert G. Ridell, and Terry Vanden L. Hoek.

5. Rachel Garfield and Anthony Damico, "The Coverage Gap: Uninsured Poor Adults in States that Do Not Expand Medicaid—An Update," Henry J. Kaiser Family Foundation, Menlo Park, Calif., October 23, 2015.

6. Jean-Jacques Rousseau, *The Social Contract* (Hertfordshire, U.K.: Wordsworth, 1998), 68.

7. For a subtle look at the social contract between patrons and peasants, see James C. Scott, *The Moral Economy of the Peasant: Rebellion and Subsistence in Southeast Asia* (New Haven, Conn.: Yale University Press, 1976), 159.

8. Jean Hampton, *Hobbes and the Social Contract Tradition* (Cambridge: Cambridge University Press, 1986), 4.

9. R. G. Collingwood, *The New Leviathan; or Man, Society, Civilization, and Barbarism*, rev. ed., edited by David Boucher (Oxford, U.K.: Clarendon, 1992 [1942]).

10. Oliver Zunz, ed., *Social Contracts under Stress: The Middles Classes of America, Europe and Japan at the Turn of the Century* (New York: Russell Sage Foundation, 2002).

11. Hans J. Rosenberg, *Bureaucracy, Aristocracy and Autocracy: The Prussian Experience* (Cambridge, Mass.: Harvard University Press, 1958); E. P. Hennock, *The Origin of the Welfare State in England and Germany* (Cambridge: Cambridge University Press, 2007); Hermann Beck, *The Origins of the Authoritarian Welfare State in Prussia* (Ann Arbor: University of Michigan Press, 2009).

12. Sarah Ferris, "Majority Still Supports Single-Payer Option, Poll Finds," *Hill*, January 19, 2015; Benjamin I. Page and Lawrence R. Jacobs, *Class War: What Americans Really Think about Economic Inequality* (Chicago: University of Chicago Press, 2009), 66. On the Republican Party origins of the Affordable Care Act, see Robert Reich, "The Irony of Republican Disapproval of Obamacare," *Christian Science Monitor*, October 28, 2013.

13. Rawls's "veil of ignorance" introduces the assumption of equality at the design stage so as to work against such skewed outcomes. If you knew you could randomly wind up in the bottom rung beforehand, how would you then design society so as to increase the odds of making your life a good one?

14. *North Shore Gas Company v. Environmental Protection Agency*, 930 F.2d 1239, 1243 (1991).

15. As early as the 1990s, the U.S. Congress Office of Technology Assessment acknowledged this difference. *International Comparisons of Administrative Costs in Health Care* (Washington, D.C.: Government Printing Office, 1994), OTA-BP-H-135, September 1994, accessed 26 October 2015 at http://ota.fas.org.

16. Bruce Bartlett, "The Conservative Case for a Welfare State," *Dissent*, July 2015.

# Repowering Chicago

## *Accelerating the Cleaner, More Resilient, and More Affordable Electricity Market Transformation*

HOWARD A. LEARNER

*ENVIRONMENTAL LAW AND POLICY CENTER*

Smart policies drive energy markets. They are spurring clean energy technological innovations that, when developed and deployed in the United States and then transferred to developing countries, can change the world through better energy access, affordability and reliability, and climate change solutions. Solar energy combined with battery storage, wind power, and advanced lighting and other energy efficiency technologies are game changers. They are disruptive technologies that will transform the electricity system just as wireless technologies have reshaped telecommunications, changing the ways we live and work.

The electricity market of the future will be driven by more pro-competitive policies and accelerating technological innovations. State and local policies should open up the century-old electric utility monopolies to more competition from distributed technologies, lower regulatory barriers to new market entrants competing on both price and services, and nudge and incentivize capital investments accelerating modern renewable energy technologies.

Solar power is making great advances through policy drivers and technological innovations. Energy efficiency improvements are saving people and businesses money on their utility bills, creating new installation jobs, keeping money in local economies, and reducing carbon pollution to protect public health and the environment. New clean energy technologies developed in the United States can be shared with emerging economies and the developing world to reduce global carbon pollution.

The electricity market is thus on the verge of rapid transformation through distributed solar energy generation, wind power development, new energy efficiency technologies, and battery storage improvements. Technological advances are bypassing the antiquated monopoly electric utility regulatory compact just as cell phones bypassed landline phones, fundamentally changing the Ma Bell monopoly and making historic telecommunications regulation mostly obsolete.

Clean energy is poised to accelerate as rapidly as smartphones, digital cameras, and wireless technologies reshaped telecommunications and changed the ways that businesses do business and how people communicate, access information, take photographs, listen to music, and share photos and information. We have learned to live and work very differently over the past two decades. For many people, a smartphone (and a laptop or tablet computer with Skype), Wi-Fi, a router, and Bluetooth internet connection have replaced the landline phones that ran into almost every home through wires and poles that lined the streets and roadways across our landscape.

Chicago can and should be a leading global city on the leading edge of clean energy policy, innovative technology development, and deployment that are a win-win for environmental progress, job creation, and economic growth, and for building sustainable and resilient communities.

How can Chicago lead? The Chicago region has the following competitive strengths and advantages:

- smart policy, business, and financial talent
- investment capital seeking new opportunities
- top engineering schools and two national laboratories
- a skilled technical workforce
- many large buildings—including commercial and industrial buildings, big-box retail stores, warehouses, schools, and multifamily residential buildings—with flat, unshaded roofs that are prime sites for installing rooftop solar photovoltaic panels
- underutilized old industrial brownfield sites that are ripe for installing solar brightfields
- old buildings with greatly untapped energy efficiency opportunities to avoid wasted energy
- national and global visibility

Chicago and Illinois already have more than four hundred solar energy and wind power supply chain businesses.[1] Policy decisions and the political will to accelerate the clean energy development transformation will make the difference for whether Chicago leads or follows.

Why should Chicago lead and not follow? Clean energy technologies will sweep the world in the way that semiconductors, wireless communications, and biotechnology have already changed our society and our economy. Chicago was late to the game as the Silicon Prairie, having missed the early game with wireless telecommunications or biotechnology. Chicago should not miss the opportunity to be at the leading edge of the global economy when it comes to clean renewable energy, battery storage, and energy efficiency technologies.

Moreover, Chicago's and Illinois's fiscal crises will ultimately require increases in Illinois's, Cook County's, the city's, and related city agencies' taxes and fees of various types, all of which will hurt many people and businesses and make Chicago less economically competitive. That necessitates that we save money in other places wherever possible. Energy waste is avoidable, and energy savings can be monetized.

Energy waste is a prime opportunity for both economic savings and environmental gains. The Chicago region does not produce coal, uranium, or natural gas. When Chicago businesses and residential consumers buy electricity from Commonwealth Edison and other conventional energy providers using centralized coal, nuclear, and natural gas–fired generating plants—and buy natural gas from Peoples Gas, Nicor, North Shore Gas, and other providers for home heating and cooking—the fuel charges are a large component of their utility bills.[2] Utility ratepayers' fuel payments drain billions of dollars from Chicago's economy to those places where coal, uranium, and natural gas are mined and drilled.

Since 2008, Illinois power producers have spent almost $14 billion on coal purchases, $11.8 billion of which was mined in other states.[3] This means that almost $2 billion leaves the state each year to import coal. Since 2008, Illinois power producers have also spent more than $1.7 billion on natural gas purchases, averaging almost $250 million each year—that amount is for electricity generation only and does not include expenditures for natural gas used for heating buildings.

Chicago's underlying utility infrastructure is also stressed. Peoples Gas is enmeshed in a very expensive and controversial pipeline replacement program extending over many years, and Commonwealth Edison's electricity wires-and-poles distribution grid—with transformers, substations, capacitors, and so on—shows signs of aging and stress in places. Repairs and upgrades are costly. Distributed generation and storage, continually improving efficiency technologies, smart-energy management systems, demand response approaches, and microturbines lighten the load on the grid and enhance reliability and resilience.

This more distributed system is more flexible, adjustable, and diverse, and less bulky, static, and vulnerable to massive disruptions and wide-scale outages. (It is also less vulnerable to terrorism and other security threats.) The improved resilience from a more distributed electricity system is even more important as climate change causes more extreme weather events that can damage and paralyze the currently centralized electricity generating system. Hurricanes Sandy and Katrina tragically demonstrated this vulnerability elsewhere in the nation.

## TRANSFORMING THE ELECTRICITY MARKET
## WITH CLEAN TECHNOLOGIES AND SOUND POLICIES

### Solar Energy Generation Is a Game-Changing Technology

Commercial photovoltaic (PV) panel efficiencies improve about 1 percent each year, and the inverters, which convert DC power from the panels into AC power that can be used for plugs in homes and businesses, have improved from 80–85 percent efficiency up to 98–99 percent efficiency.[4] PV module (panel) costs have dramatically dropped over the past seven years to between $0.60 and $0.75 per watt, and overall solar installation costs have sharply declined to between $2 and $4 per watt.[5] According to the Lawrence Berkeley National Laboratory, "U.S. distributed solar prices have continued to rapidly fall, declining by 10 to 20% in 2014, with similar trends persisting into 2015."[6]

The pace of technological change for solar energy reflects the experiences with computers, smartphones, digital cameras, remote sensing equipment, streaming music, Skype and other videoconferencing tools, and aspects of the so-called sharing economy. More than 90 percent of Americans now have cell phones, virtually all of which have been acquired over the past twenty years.[7] Over the past four years, smartphone ownership has almost doubled.[8]

The inflection point for solar energy on the growth curve is coming fast. In 2014, the U.S. residential solar market had its third consecutive year of more than 50 percent growth, and it was the first year that residential exceeded nonresidential installations. According to GTM Research, this rapid growth reflects the widespread availability and increasing diversity of financing solutions.[9]

The Illinois Power Agency's (IPA) $5 million distributed solar generation "pay-as-bid" request for proposal procurement in 2015 was oversubscribed with bid prices that a few years ago would have been viewed as very low. The IPA auction bid prices that were paid averaged $134.84 per renewable energy certificate (REC).[10] The IPA contracted for 37,082 solar renewable energy certificates (SRECs) or 7,416 a year for five years, which is about 6 MW.

If the trend continues through the subsequent planned auctions, that will lead to about 40 MW of distributed solar contracted, more than doubling the amount of distributed solar in Illinois.

## The "Quiet Revolution" with More Energy Efficiency

There is a "quiet revolution" accelerating energy efficiency through more efficient lighting, heating, and cooling technologies, more efficient refrigerators and other appliances, better building design, and more efficient pumps and motors. These continually improving energy efficiency technologies are saving consumers money and providing better service.

Rapidly coming into the mass consumer market, LED (light-emitting diode) lighting alone can reduce overall electricity demand by about 7.5 percent by 2025 in places like Chicago, as explained later in this chapter. LED lights last longer and are about 85 percent more efficient than incandescent bulbs. They are easy to install, significantly reduce electricity use, save consumers money, and reduce pollution from power plants. Federal appliance efficiency standards for a wide range of household appliances and business equipment, combined with voluntary industry actions to greatly improve efficiencies of flat-panel displays and television cable set-top boxes, among other electricity-using equipment, overall reduce electricity demand even as people use more gizmos and gadgets.[11]

But don't all of the new electricity-using gizmos, gadgets, and high-powered equipment increase overall electricity use? According to the data, no, they don't. Commonwealth Edison's retail electricity sales to its Northern Illinois customers are *declining*. The utility's weather-normalized retail electricity sales decreased by 1.4 percent in 2015 compared to the previous year. Commonwealth Edison's overall electricity sales (in GWh) for 2014 and 2015 are significantly less than in 2007 and 2010 even though ComEd has added 100,000 more customers. Electricity use is now disconnected from economic growth; put another way, the regional economy is growing, but it's doing so more efficiently.

New home and business energy management systems and smart thermostats with easy user interfaces provide control settings and automatic adjustments that dim or turn off lights and adjust heating and cooling temperatures when people are not home. Commonwealth Edison and other utilities have programs to "cycle" air conditioners to turn off for fifteen or thirty minutes during peak power demand times. Other commercial and industrial demand response programs allow customers to bid in their load reductions when that's more cost-effective than central power generation, and they can displace highly polluting diesel backup generators at peak power demand times on hot summer days. All of these technological improvements are now available and gaining an expanded market share. They help consumers save money and avoid electricity waste. What's wrong with that?

The keys here are *simplicity* and *automation*. To switch from incandescent lightbulbs to LED bulbs, people don't have to be energy wonks or tech geeks: they just have to be able to screw in a lightbulb. New refrigerators, video screens, and other appliances are fundamentally more energy efficient than their predecessors; they don't require technical adjustments by their new owner. Just as all cars and trucks are becoming more fuel efficient under federal CAFE (Corporate Average Fuel Economy) standards, all refrigerators, air conditioners and many other appliances, lighting, pumps, motors, and other business equipment are more energy efficient. As older appliances and equipment turn over and consumers buy more energy-efficient replacements, they "automatically" reduce overall electricity use and sales.

Energy management systems, including smart thermostats and other controls, have simple interfaces, automatic settings and actions, and are fairly easy to use.[12] These new energy efficiency technologies initially attract "early adopters" who tend to be younger or more tech savvy. However, as seen with smartphone, digital photography, and computer use, where user rates exceed 90 percent of Americans, these energy efficiency technological improvements will soon benefit consumers of all incomes, and older consumers as well as younger tech hipsters.

Finally, energy efficiency is the best, fastest, and cheapest solution to climate change problems. States' compliance with the U.S. Environmental Protection Agency (EPA) Clean Power Plan standards will spur more energy efficiency resources as a smart, cost-effective implementation strategy. The EPA's "Clean Energy Incentive Program" provides states with bonus allowances for early actions to install energy efficiency improvements in lower-income communities.

### Advancing Battery and Other Storage Technologies

Rooftop solar and wind energy farms used in conjunction with advanced batteries and other improved storage technologies are the holy grail that will enable clean renewable energy to mostly power our homes and businesses 24/7. There have been tremendous advances in battery improvements for computers, smartphones, cameras, and, likely soon, for electric vehicles. The batteries are increasingly smaller and lighter, more powerful, and less expensive. As GE, Johnson Controls, Tesla—which, in some ways, is more a battery company than a car company—and others seek to improve batteries for electric vehicles, there may be new opportunities for that highly distributed storage to supply electricity to homes and back to the grid when needed.

Argonne National Laboratory's "multidisciplinary team of world-renowned researchers are working in overdrive to develop advanced energy storage technologies to aid the growth of the U.S. battery manufacturing industry, transition the U.S. automotive fleet to plug-in hybrid and electric vehicles, and enable greater use of renewable energy."[13] The Joint Center for Energy Storage Research at Argonne is a national research consortium with the "5-5-5" goal of developing new battery technologies within five years to store at least five times more energy than today's lithium-ion batteries at one-fifth the cost. Tesla's Gigafactory 1, a large-scale new lithium-ion battery production plant in Nevada, is planned to be operational by 2016–17.

New home energy management systems can help allocate solar PV–generated electricity for use or for storage depending on instant market prices and priority household power needs in the same way that sophisticated trading programs guide stock purchases and sales amid changing market prices. Microgrids and new community solar gardens using distributed local generation with local storage can stabilize the grid, increase resilience by reducing reliance on extended transmission lines, and support cleaner solar generation.

### Achieving Clean Power Plan Compliance the Smartest Way for Chicago

The EPA's final Clean Power Plan rule intends to reduce carbon pollution from power plants by 32 percent by 2030. Among other things, it requires Illinois to adopt a plan to reduce its carbon pollution by 31 percent by 2030 from 2012 levels and to achieve specific interim progress by 2022.[14] The Clean Power Plan provides states with three essential building blocks for compliance: increasing the efficiency of coal plant operations to reduce the amount of carbon pollution per unit of electricity generated; moving from coal generation to less carbon-intensive natural gas–fired power plants; and accelerating renewable energy generation, like solar energy and wind power, which is zero carbon.[15] There are also some very particular energy efficiency opportunities for investment and compliance.

The devil is in the details of this comprehensive set of carbon pollution reduction standards, but, overall, the strategic implications for Chicago are clear. Investments in solar energy developments and in energy efficiency retrofits of Chicago buildings to help achieve Illinois's Clean Power Plan compliance inject capital, create local jobs, and benefit the Chicago economy. On the other hand, investments in retrofitting coal plants and new natural-gas plants elsewhere in Illinois pull money out of the Chicago economy. Chicago's policy makers and business and civic leaders should strategically focus on Clean Power Plan compliance strategies that are thus both good for Chicago's economy and good for Chicago's environment.

### Focusing on the Competitive Energy Market of the Future

Chicagoans currently choose among seven or more wireless phone companies offering varying competing rates and billing packages, services, and equipment. By most accounts, that competition and choice has lowered cost to consumers and expanded communications opportunities. Almost all Americans have cell phones and other wireless services, and as of 2013, 44 percent of midwestern homes did not have a landline phone.[16] That percentage is likely much higher in Chicago and other urban centers. Many people under the age of thirty-five are wireless-only; they either never subscribed to or discarded their landline phones long ago. As *Time* magazine titled its article on the subject, "Landline Phones Are Getting Closer to Extinction."[17]

Telecommunications companies adopted various business strategies as wireless technologies entered the market. Verizon divested and sold off its landline phone service and concentrated on building the nation's largest competitive broadband and wireless mobile phone business. Other telephone companies stuck with regulated landlines and plain old telephone service (POTS). The market results were reflected in the rapidly accelerating number of households that rely on a smartphone and laptop computer or tablet wirelessly linked to a router or directly to a cell tower instead of a landline phone connected by wires to poles to more wires and then distant switching stations. Northern Illinois has a legacy of wasted investment in telephone wires and poles scarring our landscapes. (Think about the opportunities for removing excess telephone lines cluttering up Chicago's streets, parks, and neighborhoods.)

But, isn't electricity different from telecommunications? Well, yes and no. Yes, because it's truly easier to send radio signals through the air than it is to move electrons. No, because rooftop solar panels on much more energy efficient buildings with smart energy management systems and storage technologies can become a more flexible, decentralized electricity system served by an array of competing businesses, with some offering total energy management services and others offering separate pieces of the system.

How does this affect Exelon's, Exelon Generation's, and Commonwealth Edison's historic businesses? This is more of a pricing and customer choice issue than a physical structure issue even though electricity is more complicated in some ways than telecommunications. Exelon, the holding company, and Exelon Generation, its subsidiary that owns and operates all nuclear power plants in Illinois and many elsewhere, play in the competitive electricity power market, and they should rise or fall in profitability based on their business savvy, investment choices, and ability to successfully navigate changing risks and opportunities.

There will continue to be some, but fewer, large centralized coal plants and nuclear power plants generating electricity and transmitting it through long transmission lines to the Chicago area. There will likely be more zero-fuel-cost, clean wind power generation as many aspects of wind turbine design, equipment components, and siting continue to improve and capacity factors increase, thereby lowering costs per megawatt-hours (MWh). Wind power technological improvements are leading to more efficient and economically competitive generation.

Commonwealth Edison, the electricity distribution utility company in Chicago and most of Northern Illinois, is situated differently. Since the 1920s, it has largely operated under the traditional regulated monopoly rate-of-return utility structure advocated by the company's founder, Samuel Insull. What if many Chicagoans no longer need or want Commonwealth Edison's services, just as many consumers have deserted AT&T's landline phone services? The "utility of the future" is being supplanted by a more diverse and competitive "energy market of the future."

What will be most needed, initially, is backup electricity services in case the solar panels and battery storage operating in much more energy efficient homes and community microgrids are insufficient to keep the household lights on and refrigerators running. That backup service can be provided and priced by Commonwealth Edison, just as AT&T and Comcast continue to provide landline backup service alone or as part of a package for those who still want and need their landline phone line, priced accordingly.

However, Commonwealth Edison will soon be facing competing businesses offering backup supplies from small, local combined heat- and power-generating units in basements and neighboring buildings, backup batteries and other electricity storage units, and electricity purchased on the grid. Electricity backup might be less expensive than many think because the slimmed-down, more decentralized electricity system will be less expansive and thus less expensive to operate.

More networked services connecting information and energy technologies at homes and businesses and in communities can develop along with backup services. There are multiple decentralized local electricity solutions that are becoming increasingly viable. In addition to solar PV panels and household batteries, community battery storage technologies are emerging that can provide backup or network support. Most commercial buildings have natural-gas connections, and about 85 percent of Chicago homes use natural gas for heating. Natural-gas supplies are currently robust and inexpensive. Combined heat and power, especially with effective micro turbines or fuel cells, combined with solar PV panels can provide on-site power for commercial, governmental and multifamily residential buildings, as well as providing networked or backup support for community grids and nearby buildings.

Commonwealth Edison won't be the only game in town unless the City of Chicago, Illinois Commerce Commission, and Illinois Legislature allow regulatory barriers to constrain competition. Commonwealth Edison and other monopoly utilities won't be able to keep their market share through overpriced service—they will lose customers to new competitors just as AT&T has lost Chicago-area customers to Verizon, Comcast, Sprint, T-Mobile, U.S. Cellular, Cricket, and Boost. Other companies will provide networked services and backup support, alone, or through fully packaged overall electricity supply and services.

Who will be the new competitors? Keep an eye both on more entrepreneurial energy companies and on consumer services companies such as Google, which now owns Nest Labs, markets Nest thermostats, and has enormous amounts of individual consumer and household data. "Get ready, get ready, 'cause here [they] come."[18]

## ACCELERATING SOLAR ENERGY WILL TRANSFORM
## THE POWER MARKETS

Solar energy can be a force of change as transformative for the electricity sector as wireless technology has been for telecommunications. Solar energy is a significantly disruptive clean energy resource that, combined with battery storage, is poised for domestic and global breakthroughs because of technological improvements that are rapidly changing its economic value, policy changes that are favoring its deployment and alleviating obstacles, and its high value as a peak power energy source. Solar is a distributed generation resource that can lighten the load on the power grid and increase reliability. It is available in the electric power markets at peak demand times when electricity is needed most and prices are highest. Accelerating solar energy can be a game changer for reducing carbon pollution, helping to solve climate change problems, and providing electricity at times and in places where it is needed most.

Solar energy is at a key point to fundamentally change how electricity is supplied and delivered. The Midwest is on the cusp of distributed and central-ized solar projects becoming a significant, clean disruptive technology as is already happening in California and some other states. This is a transitional time for advancing significant, systemic change for a cleaner energy future in ways that reduce carbon pollution, create more jobs, and advance regional economic growth.

The policy developments and accelerating technological improvements in solar energy and wind power are transformative. Solar panels plus battery storage is a game changer. Wind power with larger-scale storage technolo-gies and techniques is also a game changer. Solar technology efficiencies are rapidly improving the economic viability, and policy changes are driving markets and removing regulatory barriers.

As solar PV panel prices fall to 60 cents per watt, and solar businesses learn to reduce installation costs and times, the former stretch goal of $1 per watt solar-generated electricity is within reach. Illinois (especially Chicago) and several other midwestern states are poised to be a "between-the-coasts" center for large-scale solar market growth, but it won't happen easily. Many utilities view both distributed solar and centralized solar projects as a threat. They are facing the same types of choices that many businesses often face in transitional sectors: some telecommunications companies chose to move sharply into wireless and mobile communications (e.g., Verizon, which also sold its landline business), while others stayed with landline phone service. Some automotive companies are moving aggressively into electric vehicles and hybrid gas-electric cars, while others move more slowly. Some companies moved quickly into digital photography, while others continued producing single-lens reflex (SLR) cameras and film.

The force and velocity of innovative technology can sometimes be delayed but rarely stopped. Have you used Kodak Film or rented videos at Block-buster recently? Only true hipsters and audiophiles now buy vinyl discs at local record stores.

Wind power has developed rapidly in the Midwest over the past ten to fifteen years, reminiscent of acceleration in other tech fields. In 2001, there was about 500 MW of installed wind power capacity in the Midwest, and in 2006 there was about 1,500 MW. Today, there is close to 25,000 MW of installed wind power in the Midwest. Wind power development has soared, driven by technological improvements in many equipment components of large wind turbines that have increased output and reduced generating costs, supportive public policies, public and business preferences to "buy wind," and more sophisticated siting. The rapid growth in wind power–generating capacity shows a path of what can and likely will happen with solar energy generation.

Early exponential advances in semiconductor manufacturing enabled faster and cheaper computing and storage every two years, a phenomenon known as Moore's law. Wright's law refers to how progress increases with experience: because of the learning curve, each percent increase in an industry's cumulative production results in a fixed percentage improvement in production efficiency. That has happened with increased solar PV panel production and falling per-unit prices.[19] The rapid acceleration in the use of cell phones and digital cameras, among other technologies, showed hockey-stick-style growth taking off at inflection points, rather than slow, steady progress. Solar energy, following wind power growth, is moving to that inflection point for a rapid growth stage.

Some utilities and other energy companies are thinking about how to take advantage of the opportunities that solar brings for their customers, for the electricity grid and, they hope, for their investors in the competitive market. There are new utility business investments in solar companies, such as Edison International acquiring Chicago-based SoCore Energy, and others are considering how to use distributed generation as part of a smarter grid to strengthen and optimize the system that delivers our power.

While some energy companies are looking for ways to innovate and succeed with new clean technology, however, many other electric utilities view both distributed (decentralized) "behind the meter" solar and non-utility-owned "in front of the meter" centralized solar projects as a threat to their profitably. They are attempting to stall and delay new distributed customer-side "behind-the meter" solar energy generation. As a result, skirmishes are growing into all-out fights about the future of distributed solar generation in many states.

Much of this plays out in the very important but opaque regulatory backwaters where state public utilities commissions make decisions on utility rate designs, net metering standards, interconnection standards, and what is or isn't a "public utility"—all of which can be designed to advance competition among electric utilities, legacy electricity suppliers, and diverse solar energy developers and suppliers, or it can impose regulatory barriers to new market entrants.

For example, in Iowa, Interstate Power and Light (a subsidiary of Alliant Energy) attempted to protect its monopoly and impose barriers to expanded distributed solar generation by limiting their customers' opportunities to use conventional third-party purchased power agreement (PPA) financing arrangements that are helping the solar market grow. Interstate Power and Light argued that Eagle Point Solar, a small solar energy developer and installer, should be designated a "public utility" under Iowa law as a result of its third-party financing arrangement with the City of Dubuque to develop solar PV projects on public buildings. That public utility status would impose many obligations beyond the capacity of this small solar business and, arguably, including a duty to serve the 1 million customers in Interstate Power and Light's service territory.

The Iowa Utilities Board determined that Eagle Point Solar is indeed a public utility. Eagle Point Solar and environmental and clean energy groups represented by Environmental Law and Policy Center attorneys appealed the order, on the basis of its creating a regulatory barrier to competition, to the Iowa District Court, which reversed the Iowa Utilities Board's decision. Interstate Power and Light then appealed to the Iowa Supreme Court. On July 11, 2014, the Iowa Supreme Court issued a detailed 4–2 opinion, holding that Eagle Point Solar's third-party PPA financing arrangement with the City of Dubuque did *not* make it a public utility under state law. That decision sets an important Midwest and national precedent, but while the case was pending, Interstate Power and Light delayed and stalled solar energy from moving forward.

The tide seems to be turning a bit in Iowa. Following strong opposition and media attention, in August 2015 Interstate Power and Light reversed course on its proposed changes to net metering that would have constrained solar energy development. At about the same time, Pella Cooperative Electric retreated from its plan to triple its facilities fee—the fixed part of the monthly bill, or the base rate—from $27.50 a month to $85 a month charged only to customers with solar panels or another source of their own generation. Similarly, the Minnesota Public Utilities Commission recently rejected Xcel Energy's proposed increases in its customer charges.

In Wisconsin, the Public Service Commission has approved electric utilities' rate design approaches aimed at deterring customer-owned solar and penalizing energy efficiency. For example, setting a much higher base monthly fixed charge means that becomes a much higher percentage of the monthly utility bill, thereby causing a disincentive for consumers to take energy efficiency actions because the energy usage charge (over which consumers have some control) is a lower percentage of the overall utility bill. These regulatory barriers impede innovation and competition. Several electric utilities have moved to steeply raise the fixed customer charge component of residential consumers' electricity bills. The base rates those power companies charge have gone from less than $10 to as much as $65 a month, which deters household energy efficiency improvements and solar PV installations that would reduce consumers' electricity use, since consumers pay a high electricity bill regardless of their lower electricity use. We Energies, which serves Milwaukee and other Southeastern Wisconsin consumers, was also allowed by the Public Service Commission of Wisconsin to impose significant new special charges and fees on commercial and residential consumers installing solar energy systems.

These rate structure changes are designed to insulate the utilities' profits and protect the utilities' monopolies by imposing regulatory barriers to competition from consumers installing solar energy and energy efficiency technologies that reduce power purchases from the centralized monopoly utilities. On October 30, 2015, however, a Wisconsin state court reversed part of the Public Service Commission's Order in the We Energies case, holding that the commission did not have enough evidence to back up its decision to impose a monthly fee on customers with rooftop solar panels.

Think for a moment of the ironies about how the key parties are positioned here. Environmental groups, clean-energy businesses, and their supporters are pro-competition, support removing regulatory barriers, and are advocating for better glide paths to accelerate innovative modern new technologies. The electric utility companies, by contrast, are seeking to protect their monopolies by imposing regulatory barriers to impede competition, and they are seeking to extend the operation of centralized coal-burning power plants and nuclear power plants that are thirty to sixty years old and based on even older technology. Who is more aligned with traditional conservative free-market, pro-competition principles? Who is espousing more state socialism principles?

In Illinois, Exelon and its subsidiaries Exelon Generation (nuclear power plant owner) and Commonwealth Edison (distribution utility) are mostly seeking to stave off competition from clean energy, albeit with a few notable exceptions.[20] Examples of both of those approaches follow.

- Exelon leads the aggressive national lobbying campaign aimed at stopping Congress from approving an extension to the federal wind power production tax credit. This Exelon-led anti–wind power campaign is driven by the successful Illinois and Iowa wind power development (among the top five states in the nation), which competes with Exelon Generation's aging eleven nuclear power reactors in Illinois.

- When it comes to solar energy, Exelon's position appears to be largely the same. "This year, it's the wind industry. Next year, it will be the solar industry," says Joseph Dominguez, Exelon senior vice president of Policy and Regulatory Affairs. "We're just handling these subsidies piecemeal instead of looking at the problem more holistically."[21]

- Likewise, Exelon and Exelon Generation have consistently attempted to stop or weaken—put a less charitable way, "kill or maim"—Illinois legislation to modernize the state's popular statutory Renewable Portfolio Standard that boosts renewable energy, largely wind power and solar energy, as a percentage of the electricity supplied to Commonwealth Edison and Ameren consumers.

- Exelon and Exelon Generation have generally opposed efforts by the PJM Interconnection, the regional transmission organization, and by the Illinois Power Agency to advance "demand response" resources that hold down peak power demand and overall energy use. Again, Exelon's apparent strategy is to protect the profitability of its nuclear power plants by constraining competition.

- On the other hand, Commonwealth Edison has generally been working effectively with local environmental and consumer groups to design and implement consumer-funded, utility-sponsored energy efficiency programs in Chicago and Northern Illinois that save business and residential consumers money on their electric utility bills and reduce electricity use. For example, the Environmental Law and Policy Center, ComEd, and other parties are jointly implementing a new "smart thermostat" program that can produce substantial energy efficiency savings and benefits.

- Commonwealth Edison has also partnered with the City of Chicago, the Environmental Law and Policy Center, and West Monroe Partners on the U.S. Department of Energy–sponsored SunShot program, which is designed to lower "soft costs" and to remove barriers to solar energy development, for example by expediting permitting of solar projects.

- That recognized, Commonwealth Edison has generally not supported competitive distributed solar generation in Illinois despite many opportunities to do so. It has attempted to constrict net metering and has proposed new rate designs and distribution demand charges that disincentivize rooftop solar and penalize energy efficiency.

Exelon's strong opposition to subsidies for renewable energy are easily con-trasted with its strong support for continuing subsidies for nuclear power plant generation through the Price-Anderson Act, which limits nuclear plant owners' accident liability and insurance costs, and other federal financial support for nuclear power plants through favorable depreciation and other tax rules, federal loan guarantees, and so forth. As a senior Exelon executive and I humorously agreed during a panel presentation together at an energy conference, "almost everyone in the energy industry has both an eloquent justification for the sound incentives that promote their favored power sup-ply sources and an equally vehement criticism for the unprincipled subsidies for competing power supply sources."

Policy matters—a lot. Public policies open markets to more competition or they create regulatory barriers. Policies incentivize and jumpstart market penetration of innovative new clean renewable energy technologies, or they insulate and bail out old coal and nuclear power plant technologies that are otherwise economically uncompetitive with new market entrants.

## Using Public Policies to Drive Markets and Accelerate Solar Energy Innovation

Public policy choices can accelerate or impede solar energy moving forward in Chicago and Illinois. Regulatory provisions can be applied in ways that help open the market to new competitors or impede, stall, and delay new energy market entrants. Financial incentives and statewide renewable energy standards can spur and accelerate new-technology clean solar energy and wind power that the public overwhelmingly supports as part of the power mix that is supplied by utilities, *or* policies can instead require consumers to subsidize old-technology nuclear plants and coal plants.[22] Consumers have already paid off those old plants through electric rate charges over many years. Thus, some of these old plants can continue to run even when they are otherwise uneconomic in the competitive wholesale electric power market. Such key policies individually and cumulatively can make a difference for solar energy development in Chicago and Illinois.

The Illinois Renewable Portfolio Standard (RPS) was a bold state policy initiative when enacted in 2007. It requires Commonwealth Edison and Ame-ren, as the utilities acting as collective power purchasing agents for most consumers, to buy an increasing percentage of their electricity supplies from renewable energy resources, principally wind power and solar energy. The renewable energy purchase annual ramp-up ran from 5 percent in 2010 to 10 percent in 2015 and to 25 percent in 2025. A solar carve-out for 6 percent of the overall renewable energy purchased was added. The Illinois General

Assembly then created the Illinois Power Agency to assume direct power purchasing responsibilities from Commonwealth Edison and Ameren.

For the first several years of implementation, this renewable energy standard was successful in incentivizing new development as intended. However, due to changes in other energy policies involving the rapid growth of separate municipal aggregation power purchases, governors' raids on specially designated Illinois renewable energy funds, the need for longer-term purchased power contracts rather than one-year spot market purchases, and a shifting electricity market, the RPS has become less effective at incentivizing new development. The anticipated 500 to 650 MW of solar energy that would be purchased by 2015 has gone largely unrealized. Many clean energy businesses, environmental groups, and the City of Chicago have advocated that the RPS be modernized, but the needed legislative changes have been stymied by Exelon's and others' opposition.

Illinois's wind energy development leadership has been slipping (from fourth to fifth in the nation) as other states step up.[23] Solar energy development opportunities are being missed. The Environmental Law and Policy Center's *Illinois Clean Energy Supply Chain* report (March 2015), co-released with the Chicagoland Chamber of Commerce, found that more than four hundred Illinois companies serve wind power and solar energy markets, providing more than twenty thousand jobs to people across the state who are manufacturing, financing, designing, engineering, installing, and maintaining renewable energy projects here and across the region. Thirteen major wind power corporate headquarters are concentrated in the Chicago area, more than anywhere else in the United States. The report identified more than 230 companies involved in the solar power supply chain and 170 companies involved in the wind energy supply chain. The companies were identified through an analysis of data from several industry groups and then contacted individually to confirm their business supply chain role.[24]

Modernizing and fixing the Illinois RPS is a vital policy step to keep driving solar energy and wind power development forward, which is good for Illinois jobs, good for economic growth and good for the environment. The City of Chicago has a strong interest in ending the delay and moving a modernized Illinois RPS forward in an effective manner.

## The IPA's Distributed Generation Procurement

The Illinois General Assembly, in part due to the stalled RPS, passed legislation authorizing a $30 million supplemental solar procurement in 2015–16 by the Illinois Power Agency (IPA). The pay-as-bid RFP procurement was designed to be conducted in three segments: $5 million in June 2015, $10 million in November 2015, and $15 million in 2016 for distributed generation resources. (The second procurements was delayed as part of overall Illinois "budget battles.")

In June 2015, the IPA released the results of its first solar procurement, in which $5 million of solar renewable energy credits (SREC) contracts were obligated.[25] The SREC recognizes the added social and environmental value of reduced pollution benefits that accrue to all people and businesses in the form of cleaner air and water and less radioactive wastes when solar energy produces electricity. Overall, the first solar procurement was successful and was fully subscribed with new Illinois projects. Three of the winning bidders were aggregation companies submitting bids on behalf of smaller companies. Other winners included Sun Edison, Microgrid Solar, VGI Energy, and WCP Solar, the last three of which are Illinois-based companies. This first procurement was for two categories of projects: <25 kW in size and 25–500 kW in size. Contracts are for five years' worth of SRECs.

All of the winning projects must be new, installed after January 21, 2015 and, at the latest, one year from the procurement date. The sooner that the projects are installed, the sooner the companies start getting paid for SRECs.

Solar systems that qualified in the larger system category had to be identified, so it is very likely that all of these projects will make it across the finish line. Bidders were allowed to submit speculative projects into the smaller system category. About 88 percent of the SRECs contracted in the smaller system category were speculative. For those projects, the developers must identify a project within six months or forfeit their down payment.

The IPA auction prices averaged $134.84 per REC.[26] The IPA contracted for 37,082 SRECs or 7,416 per year for five years, which is about 6 MW of solar energy. If the trend continues with the two upcoming auctions, that will lead to about 40 MW of distributed solar contracted, which will more than double the amount of distributed solar in Illinois.

The average price for the larger systems (sized 25–500 kW) was $101.09/ SREC. This works out to be about $0.60 per watt, which is 17 to 40 percent of the cost per watt to install a system (assuming $1.50–$3.50/W overall costs). The average price for the smaller systems (<25 kW) was $168.58/SREC. This works out to be about $1.01 per watt, which is 22 to 30 percent of the cost per watt to install a system (assuming $3.50–$4.50/W overall costs).

Illinois should build on this distributed solar energy procurement to help drive the market and accelerate the first major leap forward of rooftop solar installations in Chicago and the state.

## Reducing "Soft Costs"

Solar PV panel costs have declined drastically from about $4 per watt in 2007 now down to the $0.55 per watt panels that Solar City recently announced.[27] "Soft costs" for permitting, interconnection with the utility, and financing are the biggest target to bring down overall solar energy costs. The City of Chicago's engagement in the U.S. Department of Energy's SunShot Rooftop Solar Challenge was aimed at these opportunities through its Chicago Solar Express program, launched in October 2013. In developing this program, the city, the Environmental Law and Policy Center, West Monroe Partners, Commonwealth Edison, and other partners focused on ways to achieve significant permitting, interconnection, and zoning improvements in order to effect cost savings for rooftop solar installations in Chicago. The press release from the mayor's office touted the benefits of Chicago Solar Express:

> This project will help transform Chicago into a national leader in rooftop solar panels. These improvements will slash wait times for solar permits. . . . The City will launch an expedited permitting process where qualifying projects can receive same-day permit approval at reduced fees. . . .
>
> Along with the expedited permitting process, Chicago's Department of Buildings has published new guidelines, outlining clear steps for general contractors to follow for designing both small and large systems to City standards, making requirements clearer and making doing business with the City easier. Significantly lowering the cost to install large rooftop solar arrays, the new guidelines update structural design requirements to recognize improvements in the design of ballasted systems over recent years.
>
> Other reforms include simplifying the zoning process by providing policy interpretation and design guidance for all solar types in all sectors and streamlining the process for connecting solar panels to the electric grid. This partnership will introduce the Online Interconnection and Net Metering Enrollment, a tool . . . [that] will enable applicants to connect their solar generator to the grid and receive credit on their bills for producing their own electricity.[28]

Illinois's interconnection standards cover the nuts and bolts for connecting a customer's solar panels or other renewable energy facility with the grid. Modernizing and updating these standards can greatly shorten the time and expense it takes for people and businesses installing solar energy panels to hook up to the grid and begin generating their own power.

Cook County is now joining with the City of Chicago, Elevate Energy, the Environmental Law and Policy Center, and others on a related U.S.

Department of Energy SunShot Initiative to further break down barriers to innovative "community solar" projects. This will expand opportunities for Chicago-area people and businesses to access clean and renewable energy choices.

A new bulk purchase program offered in Chicago reduces PV panel costs and aggregates small project installations on residential buildings. That helps achieve a discounted price for residential solar systems. Likewise, community solar gardens are emerging—shared solar opportunities for projects that enable renters or homeowners without the appropriate roof space to buy into a neighborhood solar project and use the energy.

Large solar energy companies (e.g., SoCore Energy and Solar City) as well as relatively smaller companies (e.g., Juhl Energy and Solar Services) are operating and, in some cases, looking to greatly expand their solar energy developments and installations in the Chicago market. Some offer third-party financing arrangements in which building owners essentially lease their rooftops, the solar developers finance the solar system panel costs and installation, and the financing is paid off through electric bill savings, SRECs, income from surplus solar power generation sales, and the value of federal solar investment tax credits.

Relatively simple, low up-front cost financing arrangements and other techniques, such as the Property Assessed Clean Energy (PACE) programs, in which up-front costs are financed and paid through property tax bill mechanisms, are key to accelerating solar energy in Chicago. Enovation CEO Robert Zabors also points out that some analysts are also underestimating the impact of smaller commercial and residential solar PV installations that will likely accelerate as financing and distribution options improve and as retailers such as Home Depot and IKEA offer do-it-yourself (DIY) options. DIY consumers usually don't take their own labor cost into account, so the economics from their perspective is perhaps $2–$3 per watt cheaper before incentives.[29]

Net metering is an important ratemaking approach that enables consumers with solar energy PV arrays to receive a credit for providing surplus generation back into the electricity grid at the same price that they purchase electricity from the electric utility. In essence, the utility meter runs in both directions, so customers can offset ("net") their purchases of electricity from the utility by providing solar-generated electricity back to the grid at the same rate. Net metering corrects the obvious unfairness of utility customers paying $0.12 for electricity purchased from Commonwealth Edison but receiving only $0.04 when they sell surplus solar generation back to the grid.

Moreover, the solar generation supplied to the grid is often made available at peak power use times—hot, sunny weekday afternoons—when the power is needed most for reliability and electricity market prices are highest. Studies from around the country suggest that net metering provides rough justice for solar energy producers that are supplying high-value peak electricity to the grid when it is needed the most.

Net metering provides important financial support for distributed solar generation in Chicago as well as incentivizing decentralized grid support and reliability that benefits all. Chicago consumers and the City have strong policy and financial interests to support net metering for solar energy generators in Chicago. What will Exelon's and Commonwealth Edison's positions be as the current statewide caps on net metering are approached and solar energy generation increases?

Utility rate design structures can encourage or can financially punish energy efficiency improvements and solar panel installations by consumers on their homes and businesses. Over objections from the attorney general, consumer groups, and the Illinois Commerce Commission, in 2015, the Illinois General Assembly approved Commonwealth Edison's formula rates plan through 2019. This move generally insulates Commonwealth Edison's profit margin and locks in higher rates that can either encourage or discourage customer-side solar energy and energy efficiency, depending on how the utility's charges are allocated between the front-end customer charge part of the bill (the base charge) and the energy charge component of the utility bill, which is based on the amount of electricity used, respectively. As with the Wisconsin utilities' higher base rates, if the Illinois Commerce Commission were to allow Commonwealth Edison to implement much higher monthly customer charges, that would discourage and disincentivize rooftop solar energy installations and energy efficiency improvements because consumers would pay the same monthly fixed charge even if they purchase much less electricity.

High base rates also discriminate against senior citizens and lower-income consumers—groups that tend to use less electricity—thereby leading to opposition by the AARP (American Association of Retired Persons) and low-income consumer organizations. By contrast, that rate structure rewards heavy power users in larger homes with air conditioners and many other electricity-using appliances and devices—namely, people who tend to be higher-income utility customers.

Thus far, the Illinois Commerce Commission has mostly resisted Commonwealth Edison's requests to raise fixed monthly customer charges steeply.

Likewise, in 2015 the Illinois Commerce Commission rejected the proposal by Peoples Gas to significantly increase its fixed customer charge. The commission explained: "It is patent that high customer charges mean the companies' lowest users bear the brunt of rate increases, and subsidize the highest energy users. Steadily increasing customer charges diminish the incentives to engage in conservation and energy efficiency because a smaller portion of the bill is subject to variable usage charges and customer efforts to reduce usage."[30] This higher fixed, front-end customer charge issue, or some variation, however, will likely reappear before the commission when proposed by one of the utilities.

## TRANSFORMING INDUSTRIAL BROWNFIELDS INTO SOLAR BRIGHTFIELDS

Converting brownfields to brightfields (B2B) is an innovative strategy to create sustainable community economic development, increase direct access to clean energy, and reduce carbon pollution. Transforming underutilized former industrial sites into power and revenue generating solar brightfields can strengthen cities' climate and energy resilience by reducing the load on the electrical system, which today relies on vulnerable, long transmission lines to connect large centralized coal and nuclear power–generating plants to electricity loads in the urban population centers.[31]

There are sweet spots for transformative solar energy development on blighted brownfield sites with easy grid access in Chicago and other midwestern cities. Vacant sites with good transmission access that aren't suitable for other industrial and commercial redevelopment can be converted to energy-generating brightfields by installing solar panel arrays that connect to the electricity grid, enhancing reliability and resilience while creating jobs, generating clean energy, and boosting local tax revenues. These sites can be developed into 1 MW to 20 MW solar energy projects, which are large enough to make economic sense and small enough to access the grid.

Solar brightfield developments are a strategic component of accelerating distributed solar generation for Chicago. The Environmental Law and Policy Center has preliminarily identified two hundred potential B2B sites in Chicago and a thousand potential B2B sites across the Midwest. Site evaluation will involve careful review of industrial brownfields identified in federal and state inventory databases (Superfund, CERCLA, RCRA, MDEQ, and other sources) and by local officials. The sites must be big enough to fit at least 1 MW of solar (4–8 acres, depending on the configuration), have no visible shading from buildings and trees, appear to have no other higher best-use, and gain community support.

The first step in converting brownfields to brightfields is to identify and prioritize the best sites. Many of Chicago's contaminated brownfield sites are subject to specific U.S. EPA and Illinois EPA clean-up programs. The Comprehensive Environmental Response, Compensation, and Liability Act (CERCLA) applies to some of the dirtiest sites, which are prioritized for clean-up through federal and non-federal Superfund grants. The Resource Conservation and Recovery Act (RCRA) sites are where contamination resulted from municipal and industrial waste management operations. Illinois Site Remediation Program (SRP) sites covers voluntary clean-up projects aimed at reducing contamination to levels safe enough for redevelopment. The Environmental Law and Policy Center works with city officials to analyze the cache of large, vacant industrial sites that appear to have high potential for brightfield redevelopment.

A key, necessary step to advance B2B development is to expand financing options. Solar developers need a customer with a long-term power purchase agreement for the energy supplied, available SRECs, or some combination of the two. B2B projects have no fuel costs over the project life. Modernizing the Illinois RPS—and, possibly including a B2B carve-out as the city and some legislators have discussed—and developing a more stable and predictable market for these projects to sell their SRECs will advance a viable financing platform.

The third step to advance B2B development is to remove or reduce other obstacles by streamlining city zoning policies for B2B projects; reducing interconnection barriers; and identifying local financial mechanisms to help lower the cost of capital, such as using municipal aggregation contracts.

Engaging communities to repurpose brownfield sites with new solar PV panels for clean energy production is a multifaceted win: creating installation jobs, putting properties back on city tax rolls, adding community and displacing more polluting electricity sources. There are also potential opportunities to combine B2B projects with small distributed solar installations on nearby multifamily housing and in "community solar gardens" because of lower panel (per unit) costs for the larger B2B projects and lower start-up costs because tradespeople are already doing installations in the community area.

Solar energy is a game changer for Chicago's energy future and is on the verge of potential breakthroughs. Accelerating solar energy will directly reduce carbon pollution and provide local power solutions if the right policies are established. Distributed rooftop solar generation can also lighten the load on the Chicago region's power grid and increase reliability. This is a transitional time for advancing a cleaner energy future "between the coasts" in ways that create more jobs and advance regional economic growth.

## THE QUIET REVOLUTION IN ENERGY EFFICIENCY

Electricity use and demand are now declining in the Chicago region and broader Midwest while, at the same time, the overall economy is growing. Game-changing energy efficiency technologies, including LEDs, more efficient appliances, better building design, more efficient pumps and motors, smart thermostats, and sophisticated energy management systems, are resulting in less electricity used in Chicago and nationally.

This quiet revolution in energy efficiency is saving people and businesses money on their utility bills, creating installation jobs, keeping money in local economies, and reducing carbon and other pollution to protect public health and the environment. Electricity use and sales are declining in the Chicago region because of higher energy efficiency driven by both technology improvements and forward-looking public policies. Let's consider four data points:

- Commonwealth Edison's overall electricity sales (GWh) for 2014 and 2015 are much lower than its peaks in 2007 and 2008, even though ComEd has more than 100,000 additional customers. Commonwealth Edison's total retail deliveries were 88,581 GWh in 2014 and 86,732 GWh in 2015, compared to the peaks of 93,577 GWh in 2007 and 91,889 GWh in 2008.[32]
- American Electric Power's official forecast for electricity use in its Ohio service territory is *negative*: –16 percent overall for 2014–24.[33]
- After surveying midwestern utilities, the Mid-Continent Independent System Operator shifted its electricity demand forecast from a *positive* 0.8 percent annual demand growth to a *negative* 0.75 percent annual electricity demand through 2016.[34]
- Commonwealth Edison's weather-adjusted retail electricity sales in 2015 declined by 1.4 percent compared to 2014.[35] That decrease happened while the Chicago regional GRP *increased* 2.6 percent in 2014, and ComEd added over 100,000 more customers during the three-year period from the first quarter of 2013 to the end of 2015.[36] These data have been a generally consistent overall trend (table 1).

Table 1. ComEd Year-over-Year Quarterly Weather-Adjusted Retail Electricity Sales

| 2013 | | | | 2014 | | | | 2015 | | | |
|---|---|---|---|---|---|---|---|---|---|---|---|
| Q1 | Q2 | Q3 | Q4 | Q1 | Q2 | Q3 | Q4 | Q1 | Q2 | Q3 | Q4 |
| −1.2% | 1.0% | −0.8% | 0.4% | 1.8% | 0.0% | 0.0% | −1.2% | −1.9% | −1.2% | −0.5 | −2.2% |

Source: Exelon Quarterly Financial Reports

In short, the Chicago region's and the overall Midwest's economic growth is now decoupled from electricity use. The Midwest's regional economy is growing more efficiently.

These *negative* 1.0 to 1.5 percent annual regional electricity usage reductions will improve overall economic growth by reducing businesses' electricity costs, thereby improving their bottom lines, and by providing residential consumers with more disposable income to spend at stores on their local State Streets and Main Streets. The electricity usage reductions will help achieve carbon pollution reduction goals without sacrificing overall economic growth. This enables the Midwest to transition through more coal plant retirements without creating reliability problems.

The electricity usage reductions will also help hold down wholesale power market prices. That is financially disadvantageous for owners of existing power plants but creates economic savings for other businesses, residential, and governmental electricity consumers.

Why is this happening? As the economy of the Midwest has moved, in part, from energy-intensive heavy manufacturing to less energy-intensive service businesses, this structural change held electricity use lower than it otherwise would have been. The remaining manufacturing in the region is much more energy efficient. Electricity use declined during the 2008–09 economic recession, but that wasn't just a temporary blip as some then argued. Electricity demand and use have continued to decline during the postrecession housing recovery while Chicago's economy is growing.

The 4 to 5 percent difference between economic growth and (declining) electricity sales is due, in large part, to the quiet revolution in energy efficiency—and there's more to come.

LEDs are beginning to rapidly take over the lighting market. They are 85 percent more efficient than incandescent bulbs, last longer, are easy to install, and are quickly declining in price. As explained below, the single technological innovation of LED lighting can potentially reduce electricity use in the Chicago region by about 7.5 percent by 2025. The data point is huge.

Federal and state appliance efficiency standards for refrigerators, clothes washers, dishwashers, room air conditioners, and many other household and business appliances are achieving their intended impacts. As businesses and households turn over and replace their older appliances with newer, more energy efficiency models, that steadily chips away at electricity use. It's easy for consumers. They don't have to necessarily search and choose the most energy-efficient new refrigerator, because almost all new models on the show-room floor continue to be more efficient than the previous generation.

New household and business energy management systems, including smart thermostats and other smart devices, enable consumers to use electricity much more efficiently. Simple interfaces allow them to easily and remotely adjust heating and cooling temperatures, lighting, and appliances uses when people are not home in ways that save money and save electricity. Silently and simply, these energy management systems can significantly reduce and shift electricity use, thereby producing considerable savings. Google's Nest, the Ecobee3, and Honeywell's Lyric smart thermostats control central air conditioners. German market leader Tado° launched its device to manage in-room air conditioners with a goal of reaching a hundred thousand customers in New York City by 2016.[37]

New technologies expand the opportunities for demand response and other techniques for using appliances and equipment more efficiently or when it is less expensive. For example, air conditioner cycling programs use radio signals or smart thermostats and other devices to cycle—namely, turn off—the air conditioner during times when peak power demand is high. Commonwealth Edison's air conditioner cycling program offers a monthly rebate in the summer months to consumers who agree to relatively painless short interruptions in their air conditioning use.[38] This program should be expanded. Commercial office buildings have even greater opportunities to participate in demand response markets and programs that pay businesses to reduce their cooling intensity at peak power times. There are many other such opportunities—for example, adjusting defrosting cycles on freezers to defrost at night, when overall demand is low and power prices and low, instead of during the day. Demand response programs are an opportunity for consumers to make money while enhancing reliability.

The Illinois Commerce Commission, at the urging of the Environmental Law and Policy Center and others, has directed Commonwealth Edison to address opportunities for voltage optimization. Commonwealth Edison's study of this technology's potential in Northern Illinois found it could reduce the need for almost 2,000 GWh of electricity (enough to power 209,000 homes) each year at the very low cost of less than two cents per kilowatt-hour. This produces $240 million each year in savings for consumers. The study notes that full deployment of voltage optimization would take only about five years. These large savings have thus far been bypassed. It's a missed opportunity.

Many commercial and industrial customers have become much more sophisticated when it comes to energy management using efficiency upgrades and practices to hold down electricity bills. Some businesses invest in their own retrofits, while other businesses retain third-party energy services companies (ESCOs) to finance and help them capture savings.

Public policies including the consumer-funded Energy Efficiency Performance Standards programs for Commonwealth Edison and Ameren, and the City of Chicago's and Cook County's energy efficiency retrofit programs are making a steady and sustained difference. The nudges through rebates, incentives, and other approaches for business and residential consumers to make energy efficiency improvements are taking hold and making a difference.

Energy efficiency is quietly reducing electricity use and sales in the Chicago region through the cumulative decremental impacts of continual technological improvements in lighting, HVAC, appliances, pumps and motors, and other equipment efficiencies. As consumers regularly replace their refrigerators and HVAC systems, buy other new appliances, upgrade commercial lighting, and replace old incandescent bulbs, the steady turnover results in less overall electricity use.

Next we turn to the especially significant impacts of the great leap forward of highly efficient LED lighting and more efficient appliances. They are part of the quiet revolution in energy efficiency due to policies, research labs' R&D and technological advances, and normal consumer purchasing decisions to replace old lightbulbs and to upgrade their appliances.

## LED LIGHTING—GAME CHANGER

LED lighting is a game changer. The rapid market penetration of more efficient LED lighting alone will likely reduce overall electricity use in the Chicago region by about 7.5 percent by 2025. LED lights are 85 percent more efficient than incandescent bulbs and can last up to twenty times longer. LEDs increasingly come in a wide range of color spectrums and sizes, are dimmable, and, unlike compact fluorescent lamps (CFLs), don't contain mercury.

LEDs are moving to the front-and-center position in lighting sales displays at retail stores. Trendsetter IKEA met its goal of selling *only* LED bulbs and

LED lamps by 2016.[39] The U.S. Department of Energy and Navigant project that 70 to 75 percent of installed lights will be LEDs by 2025. That simple upgrade will save consumers money, reduce the need for thousands of megawatts of central power plant generation, and avoid carbon pollution.

LEDs are taking over in the lighting sector. GE Lighting estimates that LED lighting will comprise about 40 percent of its shipments (i.e., units) in the U.S. market in 2015, and expects that to reach 67 percent of sales (i.e., dollars) by 2020.[40] GE's internal forecasts in 2013 projected a global 70 percent market share for LED lighting by 2020, a rise from the 2012 current market share of 18 percent of $66 billion.[41]

In a conference presentation in November 2014, GE stated that LED technology will reduce United States lighting energy consumption by 15 percent in 2020 and by 40 percent in 2030, resulting in a cumulative savings from 2013 to 2030 equivalent to the electricity used by 51 million households.[42] Philips projected that the entire lighting market would grow 5 to 7 percent annually in 2013–16, with the LED segment of the market realizing much higher growth. From 2011 to 2012, Philips's LED lighting sales rose by 58 percent.[43] A former CEO of Philips noted in April 2012 that he saw an 80 percent LED penetration rate in the cards and projected 25 percent penetration by 2014.[44]

The U.S. Department of Energy published a thorough estimation of the energy savings potential of LED lighting in the United States that was prepared by Navigant Consulting. They concluded that LED market share, as a percentage of lumen hours, will reach a market share of 84 percent by 2030, saving 261 terawatt-hours (TWh) annually by then—a 40 percent reduction in site electricity consumption relative to baseline estimates (table 2). This is equivalent to the capacity of roughly fifty 1,000 MW coal plants, and approximately $25 billion at today's energy prices.[45]

LED adoption in the residential sector alone—with LEDs constituting about 83 percent of lumen hours in 2030—is projected to account for 61 TWh of savings in 2030, about eleven power plants' capacity, and a 53 percent reduction in site electricity consumption. Market penetration in the commer-

Table 2. Total U.S. LED Forecast Results

| Year | 2015 | 2020 | 2025 | 2030 | Cumulative 2013–30 |
|------|------|------|------|------|--------------------|
| LED market share | 11% | 48% | 72% | 84% | - |
| Site electricity savings (TWH) | 12 | 89 | 190 | 261 | 2,216 |
| Site electricity savings (%) | 2% | 15% | 30% | 40% | 20% |

Source: "Energy Savings Forecast of Solid-State Lighting in General Illumination Applications," Navigant Consulting and U.S. Department of Energy, August 2014, at table 3.1

Table 3. LED Market Penetration Forecast by Sector

| Sector | 2015 | 2020 | 2025 | 2030 |
|---|---|---|---|---|
| Residential | 3% | 33% | 71% | 83% |
| Commercial | 8% | 42% | 69% | 82% |

Source: "Energy Savings Forecast of Solid-State Lighting in General Illumination Applications," Navigant Consulting and U.S. Department of Energy, August 2014, at table 3.1

cial sector will be similar at 82 percent, while energy savings are significantly greater, at 139 TWh.[46] The market share for LEDs in the commercial sector is expected to accelerate even more rapidly than in the residential sector (table 3).

There will be a greater reduction in electricity sales in the Chicago region through increased LED market share than the national and midwestern averages. In 2014, U.S. electricity use totaled 3,724 TWh. The residential sector constituted the greatest portion of that use (1,403 TWh, or 38%), followed by the commercial sector (1,358 TWh, or 36%).[47] In both sectors, lighting is a substantial driver of electricity consumption. Lighting is the second-largest single end-use in the residential sector (150 TWh, or 11% of residential use), and it is the largest single end use in the commercial sector (262 TWh, or 19% of commercial use).[48] Overall, residential lighting represents about 4 percent of all U.S. electricity consumption, and commercial lighting represents about 7 percent.

The potential for electricity use savings in the Midwest are even greater than the overall national projections. According to a report prepared for the U.S. Department of Energy by DNV KEMA Energy and Sustainability and Pacific Northwest National Laboratory, every midwestern state had above-average energy consumption for lighting in 2010.[49] The exact cause for this trend cannot be determined definitively without more data. However, the report notes that the Midwest has an above-average number of lamps per household (71.2–89 vs. 67.4 U.S.) and power per lamp (49.4W–53W vs. 47.7W U.S.); see table 4.

These data show that Illinois and Missouri have a combination of the highest average lamp power per household, the largest average number of light bulbs (lamps) per household, and the largest average number of incandescent bulbs per household. The bottom line: the acceleration of LEDs' market share will achieve above-average electricity use savings in Illinois, which has 15.1 percent higher than the national average number of overall light bulbs and 20 percent higher than the national average number of old, inefficient incandescent bulbs to be replaced.

Table 4. Midwestern Household (HH) Lighting Statistics by State

| | Average Daily HH Electricity Consumption for Lighting (W) | Average Lamp Power/ HH (W) | Average No. Lamps (all)/ HH | Average No. INC/HH | Average No. CFL/HH | Average No. Other/HH |
|---|---|---|---|---|---|---|
| U.S. | 4,679 | 47.7 | 67.4 | 41.9 | 14.3 | 11.2 |
| IN | 4,874 | 51.2 | 71.2 | 48.4 | 11.8 | 10.9 |
| OH | 4,874 | 51.2 | 71.2 | 48.4 | 11.8 | 10.9 |
| WI | 4,977 | 49.6 | 73.8 | 48.6 | 15.9 | 9.4 |
| IL | 5,061 | 53.5 | 77.6 | 50.3 | 16.6 | 10.7 |
| IA | 5,095 | 53.2 | 77.1 | 46.8 | 17.4 | 12.8 |
| MN | 5,095 | 53.2 | 77.1 | 46.8 | 17.4 | 12.8 |
| ND | 5,095 | 53.2 | 77.1 | 46.8 | 17.4 | 12.8 |
| SD | 5,095 | 53.2 | 77.1 | 46.8 | 17.4 | 12.8 |
| MI | 5,271 | 49.4 | 71.1 | 46.6 | 11.9 | 12.5 |
| KS | 5,353 | 51.2 | 75.8 | 46.6 | 17.0 | 12.2 |
| NE | 5,353 | 51.2 | 75.8 | 46.6 | 17.0 | 12.2 |
| MO | 6,289 | 53.0 | 89.0 | 53.4 | 18.2 | 17.5 |

INC = Incandescent; CFL = Compact Fluorescent Lamp
Source: "Residential Lighting End-Use Consumption Study," DNV KEMA Energy and Sustainability, December 2012, http://apps1.eere.energy.gov

In Commonwealth Edison's service territory in Northern Illinois, lighting is a much larger percentage of the residential and commercial sectors' electricity use than the national average percentages. The energy savings impacts of switching from incandescent bulbs to LEDs are thus even greater.

In 2014, electricity sales totaled 88,581 GWh in Northern Illinois. The small commercial and industrial sector constituted the greatest portion of that use (32,146 GWh, or 36.3%), followed by the large commercial and industrial sector (27,847 GWh, or 31.4%) followed by the residential sector (27,230 GWh, or 30.7%).[50] The City of Chicago also has a great deal of outdoor lighting.

Lighting is the largest single end use in the Northern Illinois residential sector: 5,528 GWh, or 20.3 percent of residential use, and thus 6.2 percent of overall electricity consumption in Northern Illinois.[51] This is significantly different than the rest of the United States, in which lighting makes up the second-largest end use at 11 percent on average.[52] In Chicago, according to Commonwealth Edison, residential lighting usage totals 1,189 GWh, which accounts for 19 percent of residential electricity usage and 5.24 percent of overall electricity usage across all sectors.[53]

Commercial and industrial lighting accounts for about 12.3 percent of overall electricity consumption in Northern Illinois. In Chicago, according to Commonwealth Edison, commercial and industrial lighting totals 4,599 GWh, which accounts for 28 percent of total commercial and industrial electricity usage and 20.27 percent of overall electricity usage across all sectors.[54]

For Commonwealth Edison's service territory in Northern Illinois and in Chicago, here's the impact by the numbers. The projected switching 71 percent of the lumen-hours to LEDs in the residential sector by 2025 would, alone, reduce almost 3 percent of overall electricity demand in Northern Illinois.[55] The calculation for the commercial and industrial sectors has more variables but is likely in the range of an additional 3.5 percent reduction of overall electricity demand in Northern Illinois by 2025.[56] Add in more electricity use reductions from LED installations in governmental facilities that are not included in the commercial customer class.

The projected market penetration of LEDs by 2025 is thus likely to reduce overall electricity use in Northern Illinois by about 7.5 percent from the combined residential, commercial, industrial, and governmental customer classes.

In Chicago,

- the projected adoption of LEDs in the residential sector will reduce overall electricity usage by 2.05 percent;
- the projected adoption of LEDs in the commercial and industrial sectors will reduce overall electricity usage by 5.47 percent; and
- the combined result is that projected LED installations will lead to a 7.52 percent reduction in electricity usage by 2025.

The energy savings potential of more efficient lighting technologies, especially LEDs, is thus very large and can reduce the need for central generating power plants.

Retail prices on LEDs are falling quickly and speeding adoption rates. Solid-state lighting (SSL) technology has advanced such that LEDs meet or exceed the quality of light produced by incandescent and fluorescent lamps for residential and commercial applications, while using significantly less electricity (~200 lm/W for LEDs by 2020) and lasting many times longer (~50,000 hours for indoor LEDs by 2020). The previously high price of LED lamps was a barrier to their widespread deployment. However, manufacturing advances, energy policies, and global supply chain innovations have combined to drive down prices at a greater-than-forecast rate, which is speeding their market penetration.

McKinsey and Company updated its 2011 study on the global lighting market in 2012 to show that LED package prices were declining 4 percent per year faster than expected.[57] This means that the so-called inflection point for LED lights in the residential sector—the price point at which paybacks are faster than the perceived consumer acceptance of a 2–3 year threshold—will be reached in

2015. Navigant also remarks in its study that some SSL manufacturers foresee LED market penetration occurring at faster-than-projected rates.[58]

The rapid price reductions are also referenced by several major manufacturers' public statements and activity. In January 2012, Philips announced price cuts to its LED lightbulbs, and its CEO has stated they are aiming for a price point for LED bulbs at "well below $10."[59] Cree, a U.S. manufacturer, cut the price of outdoor streetlights by 50 percent. In 2012, Environmental Law and Policy Center staff found only three brands of indoor LED lights being sold at Home Depot that were priced below $10 per bulb. In 2015, there were no fewer than eight brands of LEDs with offerings below $10.

These price drops and consumer acceptance of LEDs are occurring around the Midwest. In Ohio, for example, American Electric Power reported that although only 2 to 3 percent of bulbs sold were LEDs in 2013, the market share for LEDs rose to 11 percent in 2014.

In sum, LEDs are an easily installed game-changing efficiency technology that will significantly reduce electricity use in Chicago and throughout the nation over the next decade.

## MORE ENERGY EFFICIENT APPLIANCES—GAME CHANGER

The energy savings potential of more efficient appliances is very large. Federal and state appliance efficiency standards driven by public policies, technological improvements as appliance manufacturers compete on the basis of energy efficiency ratings, and market demand driven by the U.S. EPA Energy Star program and overall consumer awareness are combining to reduce electricity use. In some cases, European standards have also caused U.S. manufacturers to improve their efficiencies for appliances sold in global markets.

The Illinois Energy Efficiency Performance Standards program and other efficiency programs, which provide rebates and other incentives for purchases of more efficient lighting, appliances, and other equipment, nudge consumers to adjust their buying patterns to upgrade sooner (thereby gaining energy savings sooner) and choose more efficient appliances.

As of 2011, energy efficiency standards for household appliances reduced total U.S. electricity consumption by 7 percent. By 2025, existing standards will have reduced electricity consumption by 682 TWh, or 14 percent relative to usage without standards, resulting in an electricity use reduction equivalent to 114 1,000 MW coal plants.

The residential sector accounts for 38 percent of overall national electricity use. Since 1990, the U.S. Department of Energy (DOE) has periodically issued updates on efficiency performance standards for appliances ranging from refrigerators to clothes washers, dishwashers, central air conditioners, and heat pumps. For central air conditioners and heat pumps, "DOE estimates that the standards will save about 1 quad (quadrillion Btu) of energy over 30 years and yield a net present value of about $4 billion at a 3 percent discount rate."[60]

New and updated efficiency standards are continually in the pipeline. For example, in September 2015, the DOE opened the public portion of the process of bringing battery chargers into the circle of appliances subject to energy conservation standards.[61] These DOE appliance and equipment efficiency standards, combined with state and utility-sponsored energy efficiency performance standards programs, have driven greater market penetration for efficient appliances.

By 2011, the adoption of standards for energy efficient household appliances had reduced total U.S. electricity consumption by 7 percent. By 2025, existing standards will have reduced electricity consumption by 14 percent relative to usage without standards.[62] Net economic savings in 2010 were $27 billion, and by 2025 are projected to be $60 billion. At the same time that appliances have become more energy efficient, their prices have mostly declined or stayed about the same, and their quality has improved (table 5).

Another example of efficiency savings that can be gained is adjusting refrigerator defrost cycles. Defrosting refrigerators accounts for 5 to 15 percent of units' total energy usage. Many refrigerators utilize outdated, inefficient automatic defrosters or must be defrosted manually. The most simple automatic defrosters are set to defrost the refrigerator every 6, 8, 10, 12, or 24 hours, with many set to more frequent defrost cycles that are not needed. Manufacturers do not set these cycles to run off-peak so many refrigerators run unnecessary defrosting during peak electricity use times. Many customers also fail to manually defrost refrigerators on a regular basis; that requires the units to use more energy to keep them properly cooled. It is not difficult on most refrigerators to reprogram the defrost cycle so it both runs less frequently and takes place during off-peak electricity times at night.

Table 5. Changes in Energy Usage and Price of Major Appliances

|  | Base Year | Energy Usage Change | Price Change |
|---|---|---|---|
| Room AC | 2001 | −23% | 18% |
| Clothes washers | 1987 | −45% | −75% |
| Dishwashers | 1987 | −30% | −50% |
| Refrigerators | 1987 | −50% | −35% |

Source: American Council for an Energy-Efficient Economy, "Better Appliances: An Analysis of Performance, Features, and Price as Efficiency Has Improved," May 2013

Federal appliance efficiency standards and rebates and other incentives offered through state energy efficiency programs are leading to new refrigerators being replaced more quickly with more efficient ones. Techniques to shift defrosting cycles to off-peak times is an additional efficiency opportunity, especially as smart thermostats and smart meters are installed in the Chicago-area homes. There appear to be a potentially large amount of energy savings to be gained in this area through consumer education and approaches by utilities, manufacturers, and contractors to reprogram and otherwise change defrost cycle settings to off-peak times.

Televisions are the fifth-highest residential electricity use but have so far not been included in federal energy efficiency standards. However, in 2009, California, with support from manufacturers, retailers, and environmental groups, implemented the strictest energy standards in the world for televisions: 33 percent average electricity use reduction by 2011 and 49 percent average reduction by 2013.[63] These standards are projected to reduce total electricity use in California by 1 percent, and because most manufacturers upgrade all televisions to meet these California market standards, the energy savings will be achieved nationally.

The Northwest Power and Conservation Council determined that from 2009 to 2013, the average electricity use of new televisions in the four Pacific Northwest states declined by more than 50 percent, and the share of Energy Star–certified televisions increased from 20 percent to almost 100 percent. They also estimate that improvements in television set efficiency over the next twenty years will cost-effectively reduce regional loads by 390 MW.[64]

Assuming that all new televisions in the United States will meet the California standards, and that 10 percent are replaced and turned over each year, the increased efficiency for televisions alone will save about 4.7 TWh of electricity per year in the United States. Over ten years, this would amount to avoiding over seven power plants' worth of new capacity nationwide.

The electronics industry is likewise greatly increasing the energy efficiency of both flat panel video screens and TV set-top boxes. For example, in December 2013, the U.S. Department of Energy and leading manufacturers announced an agreement to improve TV set-top box efficiency, aiming at 90 percent penetration of certain energy saving measures in new boxes and software updates to already-deployed boxes.[65]

LED lighting and more energy-efficient appliances are game changers, producing significant electricity use and demand reductions in the Chicago region. This white paper, however, scratches only the surface of the available new energy efficiency technologies and techniques. Smart thermostats and other smart devices, new sophisticated home and business energy management systems, voltage optimization, and pricing signals can all significantly reduce use and demand, and achieve energy cost savings. They are all growing parts of the overall quiet revolution in energy efficiency that is changing the electricity services market.

Energy efficiency is a no-brainer for Chicago because it saves residential, business, and government agency consumers money on their utility bills, creates installation jobs, reduces pollution, and keeps energy dollars in the local economy by stemming the outflow of dollars for coal, natural gas, and uranium fuel costs embedded in utility bill payments. Energy efficiency is the best, fastest, and cheapest solution to climate change problems. Illinois and other states' compliance with the U.S. EPA Clean Power Plan standards will spur more energy efficiency resources, which should be very cost-effective and made easier with more efficient equipment and better interfaces.

## BATTERY STORAGE: BETTER, SMALLER, AND MORE CAPACITY

Advanced battery and other energy storage technologies are improving. That's clear. What's less clear are how fast, how much more capacity, the sizes and types of uses, and at what prices? Rooftop solar and wind energy farms *plus* advanced batteries and other storage technologies are game changers that will enable clean renewable energy to mostly power our homes and businesses on a 24/7 basis.

The tremendous advances in battery improvements for computers, smartphones, cameras—increasingly smaller and lighter, more powerful and less expensive batteries—indicate the promising pathways for battery storage becoming a much larger, more integral part of the overall electricity system. High-powered, smaller batteries being developed for electric vehicles by several Asian manufacturers, GE, Johnson Controls, and Tesla create a related pathway to accelerate improvements for home and business battery storage for electricity. These new batteries facilitate distributed solar energy generation to supply electricity, and for vehicles to potentially store and provide electricity back to the grid when needed.

The increased intensity of R&D at both governmental research laboratories and domestic private-sector businesses, such as GE, seeking to achieve competitive market leadership in this growing field is impressive. It also underscores the very competitive global race on battery technology and market share.

The Chicago region is well-positioned with its world-class universities, technical expertise, and research centers. The Joint Center for Energy Storage Research at Argonne National Laboratory is a national research consortium with the "5-5-5" goal of developing new battery technologies within five years to store at least five times more energy than today's lithium-ion batteries at one-fifth the cost.

Argonne National Laboratory's multidisciplinary team is focused on developing advanced energy storage technologies aimed at transitioning the automotive fleet to plug-in hybrid and electric vehicles, and enabling greater use of renewable energy.[66] Argonne's research program is a center of U.S. effort to catch up with and surpass Korean, Chinese, and Japanese battery manufacturers that started earlier. Tesla's battery Gigafactory, among others, also reflects a significant investment in U.S.-made batteries. Policy makers should be considering the domestic economy and geopolitical consequences of the United States being as dependent on China and Korea for advanced batteries, just as our country has historically depended on Middle Eastern countries for oil.

New battery storage systems for electricity link to new home and commercial energy management systems that can help allocate solar PV–generated electricity for use, storage, or sale to the grid depending on current hourly market prices and priority household and business power needs. Microgrids, and new community solar gardens using distributed local generation with local storage, can stabilize the grid, increase resilience by reducing reliance on long-line transmission, and support cleaner solar generation.

Sales of commercial energy storage batteries are beginning to grow, mostly as some large electric utilities deploy in-front-of-the-meter batteries. Data from GTM Research and the Energy Storage Association show that U.S. utilities and other firms installed 40.7 MW of energy storage in the second quarter of 2015, a nine-fold increase from the second quarter of 2014. Of that new battery storage, 87 percent is "in front of the meter," meaning the systems were installed by utilities or grid operators, while 13 percent is installed "behind the meter" by home and business owners, school systems, and military bases.

For 2015, GTM projects that 220 MW of new energy storage capacity will be deployed with 89 percent in front of the meter and 11 percent behind the meter. GTM forecasts that pricing for energy storage systems will also continue to fall as the technology matures and new markets open.[67]

But that's only the tiny tip of the iceberg. Sandia National Laboratories projects that there is more than 64,000 MW of energy storage capacity, including batteries and other technologies, nationally.[68] According to a 2015 analysis by the Clean Energy Group, energy storage systems are not being widely adopted in part because electricity markets and energy investment valuations have not yet developed mechanisms that account for the benefits of such systems.[69]

Watch as automobile companies, such as Tesla and Daimler AG (the corporate parent of Mercedes-Benz and Smart), begin to sell residential and commercial electric batteries. For example, Tesla is now selling its stackable Powerwall lithium-ion wall-mount batteries for home use, and larger Powerwall batteries for commercial customers, including utilities. Mercedes-Benz is now marketing its "private energy storage plants," knee-high silver towers each with 2.5 kWh in electric storage capacity. Owners can combine up to eight batteries, which will be available for companies and private households, into a 20 kWh system.[70] Solar installer Sungevity is also offering its customers a home battery system, made by Germany's Sonnenbatterie, to store electricity from its rooftop solar PV arrays.[71]

Does Commonwealth Edison have a role to play here? Certainly in the transition, but ComEd will face more competition than it has in the past. There *will* be a need for backup electricity supply when the sun isn't shining or a home or business doesn't yet have sufficient on-site battery storage. Commonwealth Edison is well positioned to provide that backup service at a reasonable price, which might be higher than its full-service prices. In some ways, this is what certain phone companies do in offering landline phone services to those customers who haven't switched to cell phones (less than 10% of the U.S. public) or for varying reasons still desire to retain their landline phone service. That stand-alone landline service is generally costly; some companies, however, price landlines relatively lower or camouflage its cost by packaging it with cable and other services.

Commonwealth Edison will likely be able to maintain its customers for several years through the shifts to rooftop solar PV and battery storage, and a more decentralized electricity system. Its customer base will likely erode, though, if its services are priced too high. ComEd will lose customers just as the telephone companies have lost customers to wireless providers. Other businesses will likely compete by offering to provide overall electricity services, components of networked services, or backup services, or some combination of these. This will likely be a competitive business sector by about 2025, if not sooner. ComEd will have to price competitively in order to retain its hoped-for share of the electricity market of the future.

Energy efficiency will hold down electricity demand and lighten the load on the grid. Batteries and other energy storage combined with distributed solar generation, combined heat and power (CHP), and other distributed resources will enable a more connected, networked grid and community microgrids. In short, we will have a cleaner, more decentralized, more efficient, and more resilient electricity system for the future.

## SEIZING CHICAGO'S COMPETITIVE ADVANTAGES:
## CLEAN POWER PLAN COMPLIANCE

On August 3, 2015, the U.S. EPA issued its final Clean Power Plan, which is intended to reduce carbon pollution from power plants nationally by 32 percent by 2030. The Clean Power Plan requires Illinois to adopt a plan designed to reduce its carbon pollution by 31 percent by 2030 from 2012 levels.[72] The final Clean Power Plan provides states with flexible options, including choices among mass-based and rate-based approaches, and statewide and power plant specific focuses. These compliance strategy choices affect different electricity generators (Exelon, Dynegy, NRG, Calpine, Prairie State coal plant owners) in different ways. Generators are lobbying the Illinois EPA and other stakeholders to adopt compliance approaches that minimize their own respective costs, maximize their competitors' costs, and provide competitive economic advantages for their particular resource portfolios. ("On February 9, 2016, the Supreme Court stayed implementation of the Clean Power Plan pending judicial review. The Court's decision was not on the merits of the rule. EPA firmly believes the Clean Power Plan will be upheld when the merits are considered because the rule rests on strong scientific and legal foundations. For the states that choose to continue to work to cut carbon pollution from power plants and seek the agency's guidance and assistance, EPA will continue to provide tools and support.")[73]

There are also potential opportunities for Illinois to join with other states in regional compliance plans that can essentially involve trading of carbon pollution allowances or to adopt a carbon tax mechanism. That requires the participating states to adopt similar compliance frameworks. All paths lead to, at least, a de facto price of carbon production and avoidance that will be reflected in the electricity services market.

The Clean Power Plan identifies three building blocks for compliance: increasing the efficiency of coal plant operations to reduce the amount of carbon pollution per unit of electricity generated; moving from coal generation to less carbon-intensive natural gas-fired power plants; and accelerating renewable energy generation, like solar energy and wind power, which is zero-carbon.[74] There are also some energy efficiency opportunities for investment and compliance.

Illinois is required to issue its Clean Power Plan compliance document by 2018, and interim carbon pollution reductions must be achieved by 2022. Battle lines over the state's implementation choices are likely to become clear fairly soon. The devil is in the details of this comprehensive set of carbon pollution reduction standards, but, overall, the strategic implications for Chicago are clear.

For Chicago, how Illinois seeks to achieve Clean Power Plan compliance makes a difference. Investments in solar energy developments and in energy efficiency retrofits of buildings in Chicago to achieve Illinois's Clean Power Plan compliance inject capital, create local jobs, and benefit the Chicago economy. Moving to a more distributed energy system creates many installation jobs, especially in light of the large number of energy management controls companies in the Chicago region. Enovation Partners CEO Bob Zabors points out the electrical workers training program at Kennedy-King College likely produces among the highest wage jobs in any Chicago-area community college.

On the other hand, capital investments in retrofitting coal plants, and new natural gas plants located elsewhere in Illinois pull money out of the Chicago economy. The coal and natural-gas fuel costs and other operating costs likewise drain money from the Chicago economy.

The more distributed solar generation and energy efficiency infrastructure system should result in a much greater percentage of electricity capital expenditures, operational expenditures, and avoided fuel costs staying in Chicago. Chicago's policy makers and business and civic leaders should strategically focus on Clean Power Plan compliance strategies that work best for Chicago's economy and environment.

Finally, as we've seen, solar energy, energy efficiency, and battery technological improvements, policies, and installations are moving fast. Much can happen in the rapidly changing electricity services market in the seven years between the U.S. EPA's August 2015 issuance of the Clean Power Plan and the 2022 interim date for states' initial carbon pollution reductions. The federal Clean Power Plan *is* a big step forward for national progress and for credible U.S. leadership to advance global climate change solutions. In Illinois, the cost per ton of carbon pollution reductions might be much lower than expected, however, and the importance of the Clean Power Plan for influencing change in the electric power sector might be less than the impacts of savvy public policies, new financing structures, and rapid technological advancements in clean renewable energy and energy efficiency resources.

## CONCLUSION

Chicago is on the cusp of fundamental changes in which the century-old centralized electricity system will shift to be more decentralized and

distributed, with solar energy providing a greater share of electricity supply, battery storage facilitating more solar use and reliability, and energy
efficiency technology improvements and policies significantly reducing
electricity use and demand while the Chicago region's overall economy
continues to grow. The electricity market of the future will be driven by
more pro-competitive and pro-environmental policies, combined with accelerating technological innovations, and lower regulatory barriers to new
market entrants that will compete with the current utility monopolies on
both price and services.

A more distributed and decentralized energy system will be more affordable, over time, for consumers as solar PV and battery costs efficiencies increase and costs decline, and as energy efficiency reduces electricity use and
achieves utility bill cost savings. This modern energy infrastructure system
is more resilient and less vulnerable to extreme weather events and other
disruptions. It is also cleaner and less polluting. It can be developed in more
flexible sizes and locations with more community control, local economic
value, and job creation.

Chicago can and should be a national and global leader in seizing the opportunities to accelerate transformation of the electricity sector. Innovative
technologies and approaches deployed in Chicago can be models for other
cities and can help solve our global climate change problems.

Smart public policies drive electricity markets. Technological innovations
and strategies developed and applied here, and then transferred to developing
countries, will help achieve global benefits. Effectively advancing sustainability principles and practices in Chicago can be replicated and will help
change the ways that people live and businesses operate here and throughout
the world.

## Notes

The author appreciates the assistance of the Environmental Law & Policy Center's
research coordinator John Paul Jewell and economic policy associate Jesse Buchsbaum on the energy efficiency section of this paper.

1. Environmental Law and Policy Center, *Illinois Clean Energy Supply Chain* report, March 2015.
2. For electric utility bills, the fuel charges are embedded in the electricity supply
charges. For natural gas utility bills, the fuel charges are passed directly to consumers.
3. EIA Form 923 and EIA Electricity Data Browser.
4. See SolarEdge Technologies at www.solaredge.us/ and Enphase Energy at https://
enphase.com/en-us; see slide 36 (showing +98% efficiencies) in *Photovoltaics Report*,
Fraunhofer Institute for Solar Energy Systems, ISE, at www.ise.fraunhofer.de. For

an overall perspective from 2013, see, for example, Sustainable Energy Group, Ray Darby, "Technology Breakthroughs? The Silent Progress Of the Solar Inverter" (July 3, 2013): "Ten to fifteen years ago, solar inverters were 80–85% efficient. They also had to be installed with large batteries as part of the system, which added to the cost and drained the efficiency. Then, the 'battery-less' inverter was introduced and the 90% efficiency threshold was crossed, resulting in a cheaper inverter, cheaper installation costs and more power output. Fast forward to today, and improvements over the last 5 years now allow us to install inverters that are 95%-97% efficient!" accessed August 10, 2015, at www.sustainableenergygroup.com. See also "6 Solar Inverter Companies to Watch in 2015," Greentech Media, accessed March 31, 2016, at www.greentechmedia.com.

5. See figure 2.8 in "Solar Market Insight Report 2015 Q2," Solar Energy Industries Association, accessed March 31, 2016, at www.seia.org.

6. Lawrence Berkeley National Laboratory, "Tracking the Sun VIII: The Installed Price of Residential and Non-Residential Photovoltaic Systems in the United States," August 12, 2015, accessed March 31, 2016, at http://emp.lbl.gov.

7. "Mobile Technology Fact Sheet," Internet, Science & Tech, Pew Research Center, accessed March 31, 2016, at www.pewinternet.org.

8. "Device Ownership Over Time," Internet, Science & Tech, Pew Research Center, accessed March 31, 2016, at www.pewinternet.org.

9. "U.S. Residential Solar Financing 2015–2020," Solar, Greentech Media, July 2015, accessed March 31, 2016, at www.greentechmedia.com.

10. Illinois Power Agency, accessed March 31, 2016 at www.ipa-energyrfp.com. Bids for the city of Austin's much larger solar RFP were much lower—see Tsvetomira Tsanova, "Austin Energy Gets Solar Bids Below USD 40/MWh," SeeNews Renewables, July 1, 2015, accessed March 31, 2016, at http://renewables.seenews.com.

11. "Voluntary Agreement Continues to Reduce Energy Consumption of Television Set-Top Boxes," Today in Energy, U.S. Energy Information Administration, March 2, 2015, accessed March 31, 2016, at www.eia.gov, and "Energy Efficient Set-Top Boxes Saving Consumers Hundreds of Millions of Dollars," News Releases, Consumer Technology Association, August 28, 2014, accessed March 31, 2016, at www.cta.tech.

12. The Smart Thermostat program was announced on October 8, 2015, by a host of entities, "Clean Energy Victories: Smart Thermostats," Environmental Law & Policy Center, accessed March 31, 2016, at www.elpc.org/smartthermostats.

13. "Batteries and Energy Storage," Energy, Argonne National Laboratory, accessed March 31, 2016, at www.anl.gov/.

14. "Clean Power Plan: State at a Glance: Illinois," Air Quality Planning and Standards, U.S. Environmental Protection Agency, updated August 3, 2015, accessed March 31, 2016, at www.epa.gov.

15. The US EPA's final Clean Power Plan rule states that the Energy Information Administration's (EIA) forecasts "do not reflect the decline in cost and increase in performance that have been demonstrated by current projects," and as a result, the 2030 goal for renewable generation increases from 22 to 28 percent of U.S. capacity.

Quoted in Michael Grunwald, "Hidden in Obama's New Climate Plan, a Whack at Red States," *Politico*, August 4, 2015, www.politico.com.

16. Robert Channick, "40% of Homes Now without a Landline," *Chicago Tribune*, July 8, 2014, accessed March 31, 2016, at www.chicagotribune.com/.

17. Victor Luckerson, "Landline Phones Are Getting Closer to Extinction," *Time*, July 14, 2014, accessed March 31, 2016, at http://time.com.

18. "Get Ready" by William "Smokey" Robinson Jr., 1966.

19. Jim Handy, "Moore's Law vs. Wright's Law," *Forbes*, March 25, 2013, accessed March 31, 2016, at www.forbes.com (using example of "80% Learning Curve: [solar PV] Module price decreases by 20% for every doubling of cumulative production").

20. Full and obvious disclosure: the author is the executive director of the Environmental Law & Policy Center, which is deeply engaged on many of the energy issues discussed in this white paper. The author is an advocate, not a "neutral" third party, on many of these issues, but stands by the data-driven analysis expressed herein as fully supported by facts and law.

21. Herman K. Trabish, "Utility Exelon Wants to Kill Wind and Solar Subsidies While Keeping Nukes," Greentech Media, April 1, 2014, accessed March 31, 2016, at www.greentechmedia.com.

22. On public support, see, for example, Greg Hinz, "Poll Finds Chicagoans Willing to Pay More for Clean Electricity," Crain's Chicago Business, October 9, 2012: "A new poll from a local environmental group says Chicagoans are more than willing to pay more for electricity if [it] comes from clean sources like wind and solar power. Asked if they'd favor or oppose 'receiving your electricity from clean, renewable sources if your electric bill would rise by approximately $2 a month,' 73 percent replied yes. . . . That's according to a survey of 600 registered Chicago voters conducted for the Environmental Law & Policy Center by GBA Strategies, a pollster that has worked for Mayor Rahm Emanuel and others. Just 23 percent disagreed—only 13 percent strongly—according to the poll. Voters also indicated they're inclined to go a little higher than two bucks, though by a lesser margin. Asked if they'd be willing to pay an extra $7 a month, 57 percent said yes, and 39 percent no." Accessed March 31, 2016, at www.chicagobusiness.com. The full poll results are available, upon request, from the Environmental Law & Policy Center.

23. "U.S. Wind Energy State Facts," American Wind Energy Association, accessed March 31, 2016, at www.awea.org.

24. "Clean Energy: Illinois Clean Energy Supply Chain," Environmental Law & Policy Center, March 2015, accessed March 31, 2016, at http://elpc.org.

25. "June 24, 2015: Supplemental Photovoltaic RFP Results," Illinois Power Agency, accessed March 31, 2016, at www.illinois.gov.

26. "Supplemental PV Procurement Section," Illinois Power Agency, accessed March 31, 2016, at www.ipa-energyrfp.com.

27. "Solar City Unveils World's Most Efficient Rooftop Solar Panel, To Be Made in America," Press Release, October 2, 2015, accessed April 3, 2016, at www.solarcity.com; Eric Wesoff, "Is SolarCity's New PV Module the 'World's Most Efficient Roof-

top Solar Panel?" Greentech Media, accessed April 3, 2016, at www.greentechmedia. com/articles; David Roberts, "Big Solar Is Heading for Boom Times in the US," Vox, March 10, 2016, accessed April 1, 2016 at www.vox.com.

28. "Mayor Emanuel Announces Launch of Chicago Solar Express to Drive Solar Development and Create Green Jobs: Reforms Will Reduce Costs and Reduce Permit Wait Time to Encourage Solar Development Among Residents and Developers," Office of the Mayor, City of Chicago, press release, October 21, 2013.

29. Robert Zabors to the author, email November 3, 2013.

30. "The Commission rejects the Companies' claim that customer charges must be raised to ensure cost recovery. The Commission finds that SFV based rates that assume that non-storage demand related distribution costs should be allocated on a per customer basis are inconsistent with the public policies of attributing costs to cost causers, encouraging energy efficiency and eliminating inequitable cross-subsidization of high users by low users of natural gas." Peoples Gas Light and Coke Company, Proposed General Increase in Gas Rates, Illinois Commerce Commission, Case No. 14-0224, Final Order, January 21, 2015, 176.

31. Multiple solar panels at ground level are commonly referred to as a solar brightfield. Urban brownfields are former commercial and industrial properties that have some contamination or were contaminated prior to a cleanup operation, often located in lower-income areas. Remediating these sites to enable public presence and activities can be very costly, and most large Midwest cities have many sites that, overall, cover hundreds of acres. These sites can be viable for B2B development projects.

32. Exelon's Form 10-K Annual Reports filed with the U.S. Securities and Exchange Commission for the years ending in 2007, 2008, 2014, and 2015. See, for example, Exelon Form 10-K Annual Report for the Fiscal Year Ended December 31, 2015, page 134, accessed April 3, 2016, at www.sec.gov/Archives.

33. Tom Knox, "AEP Expects Demand to Fall 16% through 2024," Ohio Energy Inc., April 22, 2014, accessed March 31, 2016, at www.bizjournals.com.

34. "OMS/MISO Resource Adequacy Survey Update," Midcontinent Independent System Operator Inc., January 31, 2014, accessed March 31, 2016, at www.misoenergy .org.

35. Exelon Form 10-K Annual Report for the Fiscal Year Ended December 31, 2015, page 134.

36. "Chicago by the Numbers," World Business Chicago, revised July 21, 2015, 2, accessed March 31, 2016, at www.worldbusinesschicago.com/; and Exelon Form 10-K Annual Reports for the Fiscal Years Ended December 31, 2012, page 127, and December 31, 2015, page 134, respectively, accessed April 3, 2016, at www.sec.gov/ Archives.

37. "The 'Nest of Europe' Comes to America," EnergyWire, August 11, 2015, accessed March 31, 2016, at www.eenews.net/stories.

38. "ComEd's Smart Ideas® Central Air Conditioning Cycling," Ideas and Advice, Commonwealth Edison, accessed March 31, 2016, at https://comed.opower.com.

39. "Becoming the First US Home Furnishing Retailer to Sell Only LED Bulbs and Lamps, IKEA Sheds New Light on Home Sustainability Practices with a Bold Move to Go 100% LED by 2016," IKEA, no date, accessed March 31, 2016, at www.ikea.com.

40. Alicia Gauer, senior manager, Communications—North America Professional Solutions (NPS) GE Lighting, to Jesse Buchsbaum, Environmental Law & Policy Center, email July 10, 2015.

41. Jaime Irick, "Long View Power Demand, Energy Efficiency Conference," GE Lighting presentation, March 21, 2013, slide 6, accessed March 31, 2016, at www.ge .com.

42. Jaime Irick, "Long View Power Demand, Energy Efficiency Conference," GE Lighting presentation, November 18, 2014, slide 10, accessed March 31, 2016, at www .ge.com.

43. Robert Van Den Oever, "LED Business Lights Way at Philips," *Wall Street Journal*, updated April 22, 2012, accessed March 31, 2016, at http://online.wsj.com.

44. Stephen Lacey, "The Path to 80 Percent Market Share for LED Lights," Greentech Media, April 30, 2012, accessed March 31, 2016, at www.greentechmedia.com.

45. "Energy Savings Forecast of Solid-State Lighting in General Illumination Applications," prepared by Navigant Consulting Inc. for the U.S. Department of Energy, August 2014, accessed March 31, 2016, at http://apps1.eere.energy.gov.

46. Id. at "Table 3.1. U.S. LED Forecast Results by Sector."

47. "Table 5.1. Sales of Electricity to Ultimate Customers" (data for November 2015), Electric Power Monthly, U.S. Energy Information Administration, January 26, 2016, accessed March 31,2016, at www.eia.gov.

48. "How Is Electricity Used in U.S. Homes?," FAQ, U.S. Energy Information Administration, updated April 21, 2015 accessed March 31, 2016, at www.eia.gov.

49. "Residential Lighting End-Use Consumption Study: Estimation Framework and Initial Estimates," prepared by DNV KEMA Energy and Sustainability, Pacific Northwest National Laboratory for the U.S. Department of Energy, December 2012, accessed March 31, 2016, at http://apps1.eere.energy.gov.

50. "Exelon Announces Fourth Quarter 2014 Results, Provides 2015 Earnings Expectation," news release, Exelon, February 13, 2015, accessed March 31, 2016, at http:// phx.corporate-ir.net.

51. "ComEd Residential and C&I Saturation/End-Use, Market Penetration & Behavioral Study," Opinion Dynamics, March 20, 2013, http://ilsagfiles.org.

52. "Residential: Energy Intensity per Square Foot" table (beta), Annual Energy Outlook 2015, U.S. Energy Information Administration, accessed March 31, 2016, at www.eia.gov.

53. Data obtained from Noel Corral, Commonwealth Edison, by Jesse Buchsbaum, Environmental Law & Policy Center, October 23, 2015.

54. Ibid.; Adam Burke and Roger Baker, "Measuring End-Use Technological and Behavioral Waste to Prioritize and Improve Program Design," Opinion Dynamics, March 20, 2013, accessed on April 1, 2016, at www.opiniondynamics.com, table 4.

55. Equation: 0.71 switch (by 2025, minus 3% already LED) × 0.85 increased efficiency × 0.786 incandescents and other non-CFL bulbs as part of average HH use × 0.062 of overall electricity consumption.

56. Equation: 27% electricity savings potential from LEDs in C&I × 12.3% C&I lighting electricity usage as a share of overall electricity consumption across all sectors in ComEd territory = 3.32% reduction in overall electricity usage in Northern Illinois. The reason why the electricity savings potential is lower in C&I is because LEDs will be replacing linear fluorescents, which are already much more efficient than incandescent bulbs. Navigant estimates that T5s and T8s together are about 90% of C&I lighting in 2015. T5s have an efficiency of 84–90 lumens per watt, while T8s are 78.5 lumens per watt. As a comparison, incandescents are 11.7 lumens per watt, while the LEDs in C&I are currently around 90 but approaching 100 lumens per watt. So while LED penetration in C&I and residential will be about the same by 2025 on a lumen-hour basis, the LEDs are replacing very different baselines.

57. McKinsey & Company, "Lighting the Way: Perspectives on the Global Lighting Market," 2nd ed., 2012.

58. "Energy Savings Potential of Solid-State Lighting in General Illumination Applications," prepared by Navigant Consulting Inc. for the U.S. Department of Energy, January 2012, 66, accessed March 31, 2016, at http://apps1.eere.energy.gov.

59. Mark Halper, "Philips CEO: We'll Cut Prices on LED Bulbs," ZDNet, January 30, 2012, accessed March 31, 2016, at www.zdnet.com.

60. "Central Air Conditioners and Heat Pumps," Appliance Standards Awareness Project, accessed March 31, 2016, at www.appliance-standards.org, and "Fact Sheet on Air Conditioner, Furnace, and Heat Pump Efficiency Standards Agreement," American Council for an Energy-Efficient Economy, accessed March 31, 2016, at www.appliance-standards.org.

61. "Appliance and Equipment Standards Rulemakings and Notices," U.S. Department of Energy, accessed March 31, 2016, at www1.eere.energy.gov.

62. Joanna Mauer, Andrew deLaski, Steven Nadel, Anthony Fryer, and Rachel Young, "Better Appliances: An Analysis of Performance, Features, and Price as Efficiency Has Improved," ACEEE Report A132, American Council for an Energy-Efficient Economy, May 2013, 6, accessed March 31, 2016, at http://aceee.org.

63. "California's New TV Energy Efficiency Standards Highest in the World," Environment News Service, November 20, 2009, accessed March 31, 2016, at http://ens-newswire.com.

64. Tom Eckman, "Progress on Improving Television Efficiency," memo to council members, Northwest Power and Conservation Council, June 4, 2013, accessed March 31, 2016, at www.nwcouncil.org.

65. "U.S. Energy Department, Pay-Television Industry and Energy Efficiency Groups Announce Set-Top Box Energy Conservation Agreement," press release, Appliance Standards Awareness Project, accessed March 31, 2016, at www.appliance-standards.org.

66. Argonne National Laboratory, "Batteries and Energy Storage," accessed May 23, 2016, at http://www.anl.gov/energy/batteries-and-energy-storage.

67. "U.S. Energy Storage Monitor, Q2 2015: Executive Summary," GTM Research and the Energy Storage Association, September 2015, accessed March 31, 2016, at http://energystorage.org, and Daniel Cusick, "Electricity: Sales of Energy Storage Batteries Take Off as Utilities Try to Smooth Power Demands on the Grid," E&E Publishing, May 28, 2015, accessed March 31, 2016, at www.eenews.net.

68. Jim Eyer and Garth Corey, "Energy Storage for the Electricity Grid: Benefits and Market Potential Assessment Guide: A Study for the DOE Energy Storage Systems Program," Sandia National Laboratories, SAND2010-0815, February 2010, accessed March 31, 2016, at www.sandia.gov.

69. Seth Mullendore, "Energy Storage and Electricity Market: The Value of Storage to the Power System and the Importance of Electricity Markets in Energy Storage Economics," Clean Energy Group, August 2015, accessed March 31, 2016, at www. cleanegroup.org.

70. Benjamin Hulac, "Autos: Following Tesla, Daimler Enters the At-Home Battery Space," E&E Publishing, June 11, 2015, accessed March 31, 2016, at www.eenews.net.

71. David R. Baker, "The Battery Age Begins: Sungevity Pairs Home Solar with Batteries," *San Francisco Chronicle*, April 29, 2015, accessed March 31, 2016, at www.sf-chronicle.com; and Sungevity, "Sungevity and Sonnenbatterie Announce Partnership to Offer Home Energy Storage to Customers in the U.S. and Europe," PR Newswire, April 29, 2015, accessed March 31, 2016, at www.prnewswire.com.

72. Environmental Protection Agency, "Clean Power Plan: State at a Glances: Illinois," accessed May 23, 2016, at https://www3.epa.gov/airquality/cpptoolbox/illinois.pdf.

73. U.S. Environmental Protection Agency, "Clean Power Plan for Existing Power Plants," accessed April 1, 2016, at www.epa.gov.

74. EPA Clean Power Plan Final Rule (August 3, 2015), accessed March 31, 2016, at www.epa.gov.

# Energy Networks

## *How Do We Power a City?*

DISCUSSANT: CYNTHIA KLEIN-BANAI
UNIVERSITY OF ILLINOIS AT CHICAGO

The concept of the social contract was formulated before the electricity grid was conceived and power became a common commodity in the United States. In the many countries that still lack reliable electricity, new energy innovations are already creating a different type of power grid, much as the wireless communication technologies changed the way developing countries created phone networks. Some questions about energy that can be asked in the framework of the UIC Forum are the following: How does the social contract apply to energy supply? What is the obligation of the government to provide or regulate energy services? What is the role of the individual in consuming energy? How is that changing in the twenty-first century with technology and innovation?

The social contract for energy could be described as the obligation of a government to provide individual residences, businesses, and organizations with reliable, accountable, and affordable energy sources (for electricity, heating and cooling) or regulate its provision. In the twenty-first century, energy is seen as a basic societal need just like shelter and food. Providing that energy in a sustainable way that meets the needs of the present generation, while not adversely impacting the ability of future generations to meet that need, should be part of the social contract. Making it possible for all residents to have adequate energy to power their refrigerators and stoves, and to regulate the temperature of their homes, is a necessity.

Developed in the 1930s, the first regulatory compact for electricity in the United States created a natural monopoly service as the best way to provide electricity. This was done as investor owned, as a municipal utility, or as a co-op. Utilities would provide electric service to all consumers within their territory, and each utility would get a return on its investments that also accounted for the risks it took in ensuring service and reliability. Regulation was delegated to state commissions. This state-based approach created silos between states with respect to the national grid but provided efficiencies to the organization for maintenance of system reliability. Environmental impacts and customer choice were not part of the concerns.[1]

As early as 1997, states began enacting renewable energy portfolio standards, resulting in thirty states now requiring at least 20 percent of energy to be sourced from renewables.[2] Also, many states are deregulating the electricity supply market. This has led to more interstate discussions and to regulations designed to incentivize utilities to invest in the smart grid. This includes variable pricing schemes and the ability to sell energy back to the grid. All of this enables a plethora of innovative energy technologies on both the supply and demand sides to integrate more smoothly into the electricity grid.

Regulation of hazardous air pollutants that result from energy generation have been governed by the Clean Air Act, which when passed in 1970 set ambient air quality standards to protect public health and public welfare.[3] Using its authority under the Clean Air Act, the EPA released its Clean Power Plan in 2015 to reduce carbon pollution while maintaining energy reliability and affordability, creating the first national carbon standards. Fossil fuel–fired power plants make up 31 percent of U.S. total greenhouse gas emissions. The plan aims to reduce carbon emissions by 32 percent, sulfur dioxide emissions by 90 percent, and nitrogen dioxides by 72 percent below 2005 power plant levels by 2030. This will result in net climate and health benefits of $26 billion to $45 billion, with significant public health outcomes (annual reductions of 3,600 premature deaths, 1,700 heart attacks, and 90,000 asthma attacks).[4]

Residents, or consumers of energy, also are part of the social contract for energy. They need to contract for services, pay their bills on time, or work with the utilities to set up payment plans. They are responsible for using energy wisely if they have limited resources, and even if they don't. In other words, no one should be wasteful, even if they have the financial means to pay for as much energy as they care to use. Using energy wisely may involve retrofitting their apartment, house, property, business, or facility, all of which may be supported by federal, state, and utility incentives. Informed decision makers can purchase energy-efficient appliances and vehicles, and even choose energy providers and when to use energy. These choices assist consumers in several important ways: they keep consumers' costs down as well as reduce their demand for energy, thereby helping consumers uphold the intergenerational sustainability compact.

Energy supply has impact on two other aspects of the social contract discussed at this forum: health and environment. However, it should be noted that the United States has an inherently high-energy and high-carbon infrastructure. The average annual carbon footprint for a U.S. resident is nearly 19 metric tons of carbon dioxide equivalents, whereas the average footprint for a European resident is 8 tons of carbon dioxide equivalents.[5] Stated another way, the United States accounts for 4 percent of the world's population yet produces 25 percent of its greenhouse gases. This simple comparison demonstrates how the energy infrastructure of a country directly impacts the energy use, and that usage does not entirely fall on consumer choice.

What then is the obligation of a city, region, or nation to create a low-carbon and low-energy infrastructure? Many factors affect the carbon intensity of infrastructure: population density, climate, availability of renewable energy, and the energy grid itself. The smart grid is a key piece of infrastructure that will enable renewable energy like solar, wind, and geothermal sources to connect to the grid. Globally, we are behind other developed countries in implementing these technologies.[6] On the other hand, it was pointed out during the UIC Forum panel discussion that, for developing countries, implementing renewable energy is accelerating electricity provision—this is true because renewable energy does not require the robust infrastructure of power plants and transmission lines that developed countries have invested heavily in.

Howard Learner argues in his paper that the energy grid is changing with the growth of solar energy, energy efficiency, energy storage, and the EPA's Clean Power Plan. A key enabler of energy efficiency is the smart grid. This is a system of electronic meters (so-called smart meters) that allow for two-way communication between the utility and the consumer, ideally creating the ability to have real-time data regarding energy consumption, costs, and the functionality of the system. The utility will know where there are power outages and can reroute electricity through the system and repair power outages, quickly enhancing reliability. The consumer can be informed of price increases and respond by reducing their demand when prices are high. This produces environmental and economic benefits: since the dirtier coal-fired plants are generally used for peak-time electricity production, limiting the hours they are in operation reduces emissions.[7]

The smart grid allows the consumer to act as a supplier and to participate in demand response. When demand is high, costs increase. Consumers can take advantage of this new energy grid by using apps on their mobile devices that alert them when prices are higher. Through the apps, the consumer can then remotely power down or off household appliances—furnaces, air conditioners, dishwashers, washing machines, driers, televisions, and so on—in response to grid demand and price information. In addition, this grid more readily allows for individuals to be power providers through distributed solar, wind, and even energy storage (e.g., via electric vehicle batteries), resulting in more opportunities for cleaner energy and demand response. All of this together is creating a revolution in energy similar to what we've seen in the communications industry and wireless technology.[8]

There are several aspects that haven't yet been considered about the revolution in energy described by Howard Learner, especially as it relates to the social contract for energy. Not all consumers have an equal ability to access the benefits of the new grid. Investments in energy efficiency and renewable energy systems require capital expenditures. Although the new energy grid provides an economic payback, the capital investment needed to take full advantage of these benefits is high for many consumers. Thus purchases for more efficient and "smart" appliances will not be made for the sake of efficiency—most low-income consumers will wait until they no longer work and can't be repaired. This is all the more true for larger and longer-term investments such as for renewable installations like home solar or purchasing an electric vehicle. Those with limited resources cannot make the needed investments (purchases) unless heavily subsidized. Also, low-income households are often renters who may not have a heating or electric bill separate from their rent bill; such renters do not have a direct incentive to participate in energy efficiency or demand response. Likewise, many government facilities and large institutions, including universities, have relatively little control over energy consumption by employees, students, and other occupants of their facilities. In those situations, the occupant does not directly incur the cost of energy consumption, thus there is no buy-in, no financial incentive to conserve.

In particular, with the implementation of smart-grid technology, adoption by consumers has been slow. Only three states currently have implemented large roll-outs of this advanced metering infrastructure (AMI)—Texas, California, and Illinois. Illinois is the only state doing marketing and education through an independent third party rather than by the utility: the Illinois Science and Energy Innovation Foundation (ISEIF). The goal of the ISEIF is to help educate consumers, particularly hard-to-reach populations, about the benefits of the smart grid. The discussion at a September 2015 meeting of ISEIF grantees centered around three challenges to consumer uptake: data translation, widespread adoption, and universal access. Smart meters generate a lot of data that must be translated into dollars rather than energy in order for the general public to understand what it means and motivate them to use the data to their full benefit. The most reasonable path to accomplish this is to integrate the information into resources consumers already know: getting people to adopt smart-grid technology requires developing apps and approaches that consumers are already familiar with or inclined to use—otherwise, only the tech savvy will use them. Providing universal access through translation to many languages and making the apps or access points affordable or free to low-income users is key to widespread adoption and universal access. Much of this technology has an economic benefit to the developer and comes at a price to the consumer, a gap that nonprofit organizations can help bridge.[9]

A second consideration around energy technology and innovation is that energy is invisible to most users. Most residential energy consumers don't "see" their energy. In the past, people used wood and coal to heat their homes and cook, so they saw and even handled the source of their power. Now, energy flows invisibly to most of our households. Some rural areas still use oil, gas tanks, or wood, but such energy sources are rare in urban areas.

A third consideration is whether there is a measurable impact of energy conservation behaviors on home energy consumption and how broadly people engage in that behavior. The smart grid provides energy feedback through near real-time or real-time energy reporting. This feedback is meant to drive energy-minded behavior, either to conserve or delay usage to avoid high peak-time costs. Most energy saved through household energy feedback programs results from changes in behavior (4–12% overall).[10] Similar to the argument Howard Learner presents, others have argued that the utilization of technology will provide greater energy savings benefit than behavior change. Automated or semiautomated consumption controls would likely decrease consumption more than behavior change informed by pricing. Privacy concerns present a major challenge to the technological approach: do these technologies infringe on individual sovereignty, since they will need to "learn" about household energy behavior from the data and then propose or actually implement conservation interventions? As smart-grid technologies are increasingly adopted by society and become the norm, those privacy concerns may be diminished.[11]

The panel discussion and Learner's paper focused on Chicago. However, a brief look at the global energy picture is warranted. The advent of wireless technology provided phones for parts of the world with undeveloped telecommunications infrastructure. In the same way, renewable energy is providing access to electricity without the need for huge infrastructure. Wind and solar, paired with energy storage, can bring electricity to even the most remote areas. Developing countries such as China could benefit from a smart grid and renewable energy, but government policy must drive those changes.

Where does the less-carbon-intensive Europe stand with regard to the smart grid? The European Union adopted the Third European Energy Liberalization Package with the goal of installing "intelligent metering systems" in 80 percent of households by 2020. However, consumer demand for the smart grid–based services will grow at a slow rate without targeted marketing campaigns to enhance consumer awareness.[12]

The greatest driving force of climate change is fossil fuel combustion for energy. As a global issue, climate change calls for global solutions. We can look to the United Nations Framework Convention on Climate Change (UNFCCC), which was adopted in 1992 at the Rio de Janeiro Earth Summit. This framework is a universal convention of principle that acknowledges the existence of human-caused climate change and gives industrialized countries the major responsibility for combating it. The Conference of the Parties (COP) is the convention's decision-making body. For two weeks in November and December 2015, the U.N. Climate Change Conference (COP21/CMP11) was held in Paris. The goal is to achieve a universal, legally binding climate agreement to ensure that our planet remains a healthy environment for us to live in by achieving a less than 2 degree Celsius ceiling on global warming. Forty thousand participants including national delegates, observers, and civil society members attended. Developed-country participants should take the lead with absolute emission reduction targets. The agreement points to financial incentives that might be obtained through a carbon tax or cap and trade system that would enable developing countries to fight climate change and promote fair and sustainable development.[13] With this global agreement in place and the United States as a party to it, all of the approaches to energy—efficiency, renewables, storage, and policy—will be critical to driving the United States to lower carbon emissions.

In the United States, buildings contribute to 39 percent of our carbon emissions and 70 percent of our electricity load. This chapter has focused on the electric grid, but the topic of energy is broader. The energy used to power vehicles, most commonly through gasoline or diesel, results in 30 percent of U.S. carbon emissions.[14] Regulation has increased the efficiency of these vehicles through fuel economy standards.[15] These standards leave room for consumer choice, but ultimately the vehicle infrastructure is improving in efficiency and has reduced U.S. demand for gasoline.

In conclusion, the social contract as it applies to energy has evolved from one that empowered the utilities to one that is mostly empowering the consumer with the implementation of a smart grid, new technology, and innovation. It will require a more informed public and will call for changes that make energy "visible" to all. The increased efficiency and opportunities for renewable and distributed energy will reduce the carbon intensity of the grid, which will have health and environmental benefits. We can achieve global climate goals only through infrastructure efficiency improvements, technology, innovation, and consumer participation.

### Notes

1. "The Smart Grid: An Introduction," U.S. Department of Energy, prepared by Litos Strategic Communication under contract No. DE-AC26-04NT41817, subtask 560.01.0, undated, http://energy.gov, accessed December 21, 2015.

2. Jocelyn Durkay, "State Renewable Portfolio Standards and Goals," National Conference of State Legislatures, www.ncsl.org/research, accessed March 20, 2016.

3. "Summary of the Clean Air Act," U.S. Environmental Protection Agency, updated November 17, 2015, www2.epa.gov, accessed October 21, 2015.

4. Section 111 of the Clean Air Act lays out approaches for new and existing sources. "Fact Sheet: Overview of the Clean Power Plan: Cutting Carbon Pollution from Power Plants," United States Environmental Protection Agency, updated September 6, 2015, www2.epa.gov, accessed October 21, 2015.

5. "Each Country's Share of CO2 Emissions," Union of Concerned Scientists, revised November 18, 2014, www.ucsusa.org, accessed March 20, 2016.

6. Ibid.

7. "Smart Grid," Office of Electricity Delivery & Energy Reliability, U.S. Department of Energy, http://energy.gov, accessed March 20, 2016.

8. Ibid.; H. A. Learner, "Repowering Chicago: Accelerating the Cleaner, More Resilient and More Affordable Electricity Market Transformation," paper presented at the UIC Urban Forum, Chicago, Illinois, August 26, 2015.

9. "Mind the Gaps: Evolving Energy in Illinois," Illinois Science and Energy Innovation Foundation (ISEIF) conference, Chicago, Illinois, September 30, 2015.

10. Karen Ehrhardt-Martinez, "Changing Habits, Lifestyles and Choices: The Behaviours that Drive Feedback-Induced Energy Savings," 2011, http://web.stanford.edu, accessed March 20, 2016.

11. S. M. Stern, "Smart-Grid: Technology and the Psychology of Environmental Behavior Change," *Chicago-Kent Law Review* 86, no. 1 (2011), article 7, http://scholarship.kentlaw.iit.edu, accessed March 20, 2016.

12. E. Giglioli, C. Panzacchi, and L. Senni, "How Europe Is Approaching the Smart Grid," McKinsey & Company, 2010, www.mckinsey.com, accessed March 29, 2016.

13. United Nations Framework Convention on Climate Change, Paris Agreement Paris, November 30 to December 12, 2015, www.cop21.gouv.fr/en, accessed March 22, 2016.

14. "Buildings and Climate Change," U.S. Green Building Council, undated, http://unfccc.int, accessed March 20, 2016.

15. "Fuel Economy," U.S. Environmental Protection Agency, updated November 9, 2015, www3.epa.gov/fueleconomy/index.htm, accessed October 21, 2015.

# PART THREE
# SYNTHESIS

# Health, Energy, and the Environment

## *We Are All in This Together*

MEGAN HOUSTON

*UNIVERSITY OF ILLINOIS AT CHICAGO*

Cities are the heartbeat of modern society. The 2015 UIC Urban Forum facilitated discussions around the social contract in terms of the issues we face, and will continue to face, in urban areas. As most of the world's population is concentrated in urban areas (see David Perry and Natalia Villamizar-Duarte's chapter in this book), cities are not only where we will find people but are also where we will find the greatest opportunities for social change. Throughout the day's discussions, participants focused on three frameworks for addressing the urban social contract: health, energy, and the environment. Conversations around the roles of government, businesses, and individuals in upholding their responsibilities to society highlight the interconnectedness of each of these frameworks. Responsible energy use helps to maintain the quality of the environment, which allows us to live a more healthy life. The first panel of the day, "Rebalancing the Scales: A New Social Contract for Health, Energy, and the Environment," addressed the broader question of the social contract, and society's need to achieve this important balance. The second panel, "The Great Lakes: At the Crossroads of Health, Energy, and the Environment," brought the conversation into our very region, examining how the social contract impacts health, energy, and the environment in the Great Lakes region. Whether speaking in a broader context, or at a regional level, the conversations of remaking the social contract revolved around how all actors have their own roles to play in the fulfillment of the social contract, but all are still interconnected and share a common interest. Success will result when we are able to coordinate each of our various roles into effective collaborations and partnerships. Equally important to our partnerships is designating and enforcing appropriate accountability in upholding our responsibilities.

## ASSURING WELLNESS BEYOND HEALTH CARE

We all have our own roles to play in the social contract. The average person may not think of himself or herself as a participant in the social contract, but nonetheless, as members of society we all have a responsibility to one another. Individuals are not the only actors; the government, private enterprises, educational, medical, and religious institutions are all seeing their roles in the social contract evolve.

John Lumpkin, senior vice president of the Robert Wood Johnson Foundation, acknowledged that "most individuals don't really think about health, and certainly don't think about governmental health or public health." Our public health may too often be taken for granted when we are able to eat at a restaurant without getting sick, but we also see a heightened level of concern when we face crises such as Ebola or the H1N1 virus. Members of the public see the government as being responsible for addressing our health concerns, but they may not have a full understanding of their own role in the social contract.

Speaking to the wide variety of responsibilities assumed throughout a community to ensure health and safety, Jay Shannon, CEO of the Cook County Health and Hospitals System (CCHHS), pointed out the evolution of the school system's role in the social contract beyond its charge with formal education. Increasingly, students and their parents are relying on schools as a provider of health and wellness—through receiving medical attention from the school nurse, reliably providing a meal, and providing after-school care services. He noted that one of the challenges educators face is figuring out where their role ends. This evolution is giving schools the opportunity to engage in community-based health practices but is also placing much of the responsibility to protect the health of the children in the community on a single school. Similarly, health care systems are facing the same issue of having a responsibility to deliver care, but also a growing necessity to raise the education level of the public on health issues. Shannon sees the "blurring of responsibilities" between the health system's responsibility to educate, and the school system's responsibility to protect health and wellness, as well as the role of other social agencies, such as housing, to play a role in the health of the community.

Enactment of the Affordable Care Act (ACA) has also impacted how health care is administered in communities. Shannon explained how the implementation of the ACA has led to a shift from the Cook County health care system often being a last resort for the uninsured, to the majority of the population served having health insurance. As an organization, Cook County has been faced with trying to enhance patients' experience when they seek care. Ensuring access to care for the newly insured means being able to accommodate working poor populations. For example, offering flexible access to health services and clinics during nonbusiness hours can better allow Cook County to take care of the patients it serves. Despite progress, 35 to 40 percent of adults in Illinois are still uninsured. In providing health services to these uninsured populations, Cook County faces the challenge of ensuring that everyone is cared for in the same way.

This expanding access is one way to help ensure better health care, but there must be some education that comes along with the access. LaMar Hasbrouck, executive director of the National Association of County and City Health Officials, emphasized how there is more to becoming healthy than simply having a health insurance card. Patients need to be taught when and how to use these cards, and they may need guidance to find physicians and make their appointments. Second, having access to the necessary care does not ensure a patient is living in a healthy environment. He offered the example of an asthmatic child who has several life-threatening attacks and is able to access treatment for his asthma attacks, but inevitably returns to the same home where there may be hazardous sources for his asthma, such as mold, dust, or dander. Here, the social contract would call to engage a community health worker to visit the house and identify these health hazards in order to remediate the problems and create a safer living environment. With this question of roles and social contract comes questions of social equity, social justice, and social determinants in terms of health. Hasbrouck emphasized the importance of focusing "upstream" on preventative measures and the different social determinants that are leading to health problems in our communities. While the provision of health care services is important, identifying the factors that are causing poor health are even more important in terms of the social contract. However, the importance of access to health insurance should still not be underestimated. Studies have consistently shown that those with health insurance tend to live healthier lives. The ACA has made the first steps in ensuring that more people have health insurance, but the social contract comes into play in the broader sense of connecting the newly insured with the appropriate access to the care they need to create a healthy society.

Balancing individual rights with collective needs is always the bane of the social contract. In the context of vaccinations, and epidemic scares such as

Ebola or the H1N1 virus, Hasbrouck stressed the importance of connectedness and the concept that a single infected person in a community puts the entire community at some risk. Even those who are able to secure the best care for themselves are not exempt from bearing the social costs involved in caring for those without the same kind of access to care. Hasbrouck explained that there is the need to "balance the collective good with individual behaviors because we are all at some risk."

The recent question around vaccines is an especially important one. Even common flu shots are crucial to helping protect against large-scale outbreaks of influenza. In Shannon's view, individuals often operate under the assumption that various institutions, especially schools and hospitals, constitute safe places. Individuals, then, have the capacity to act in a manner that protects them by getting vaccinated, and the compounded effects on a larger scale will also help to protect the community. An individual may have the right to decline a vaccine, but no one has the right to infect the people around them. As a society, we must acknowledge our responsibility to one another and the impacts our actions have on our communities. Lumpkin presented the idea that too many of our discussions around health crises are happening exclusively on the national level. Without more localized discussions, the reality of social problems may not be as well understood by community residents, nor is it possible to easily inspire change within a single community. He stated that "if we are going to make progress, we really have to bring the conversations down to a community where people really identify with their neighbors." In the same way, the social contract comes into play at this local level by ensuring that individuals who are vaccinated are protecting not only themselves but also the rest of the community. We must rely on communities to get this message across because people are able to relate to their communities more personally than to national politics.

Private businesses have their own roles to play in the social contract. During the second morning panel focusing on the Great Lakes, Henry Henderson, director at the Midwest Program of the Natural Resources Defense Council, discussed the large footprint that large oil companies like Enbridge leave on our environment. The reality for such companies is, as Henderson put it, that "the business of business is business," and their interests and responsibilities to their investors should not be molding the social contract. Society's role and the responsibilities of government agencies are to focus resources on groups who are promoting the health and well-being of communities and who are invested in the social implications of their actions. It is up to us as a society to hold these companies to our own standards in order to protect ourselves.

## WORKING FOR WELLNESS IN OUR SHARED ENVIRONMENT

Collaborative relationships are the core of the social contract. All the players cannot fill all the roles, and a well-rounded society relies on diverse actors coming together like pieces to a puzzle. As with the social contracts required to assure health and wellness, protecting our environment depends on all members of society doing their part. In recent years, growing concerns over global climate change have shifted the discourse about the environment to a more united cause. No singular effort can reverse the effects of global climate change, but joined efforts among many nations' governments to manage the well-being of their peoples, and natural resources will benefit everyone. Shannon noted that "it is very hard to take care of everyone the same way." Cook County hospitals, for example, have arrived at the important realization that improvement will come only through collaboration and partnerships. Historically, when a health system was unable to provide the necessary care to a patient, a physician had no further avenues to find care for a patient. Shannon explained that today we are better able to recognize that a single physician does not possess the necessary "expertise to provide the whole spectrum of care," but by developing a network of different providers that do offer other services, Cook County is better able to serve its patients. Among the partnerships sought by Cook County are those with community-based social agencies that support behavioral health issues. By learning to partner with other organizations, Cook County has been able to broaden its services and see more successful outcomes. New initiatives from the Affordable Care Act (ACA), such as the Center for Medicare and Medicaid Innovation, which provides State Innovation Model (SIM) Grants that are not just tied to the provision of services, but that go toward improving health in other ways. For example, SIM Grants can be used to help health systems partner with local housing agencies in order to provide safe transitional housing to patients. This kind of collaboration will help protect the homeless populations against the dangers that could lead to them utilizing more health services or emergency rooms.

Recognizing the importance of collaborative partnerships is crucial to the social contract but may not always be pragmatic. Entities and organizations have an innate interest in looking out for themselves, but they also need to recognize their responsibility to others. Forming partnerships is a choice to be made by each organization, and by their nature, collaborations will require compromise. Although compromise is not always easy, it is sometimes necessary in order to sustain the social contract. When addressing policy concerns about health, the environment, and energy, it is dangerous to assume that finding and implementing a solution is someone else's responsibility. In seeking policy solutions, we too often defer to finding a specific answer, instead looking for the narrow "either/or" solution and not enough for a "yes-and" solution. Equally important in seeking solutions and cooperation is maintaining confidence in the abilities of partners. Progress will not come through undermining the competency of institutions; further, doubt will only create distrust, so we must be confident in our capacity to work together.

Henderson especially fears that the language around the dysfunction of government is corrosive to the social contract and to the potential for cooperation. We cannot have a social contract without a governing structure, and, as he said, "a good government structure reflects a solid social contract." Our modern discourse that government is a dysfunctional and incompetent external force on policy undermines critical elements of what we think of as a social contract and prohibits the government from playing its role. Henderson believes that this current language around government is "a corrosive factor that we have to fundamentally rebut." We need to recognize that federal actions, such as the Clean Air Act (CAA), Clean Water Act (CWA), and the formation of the Environmental Protection Agency (EPA), have had the power to bring about positive policy changes that have had great impacts on people's lives. We should not dismiss government action as hopeless, because its role is key to maintaining the social contract.

Lumpkin emphasized the significance of rejecting these negative outlooks, citing the myth that it isn't economically viable for major chain grocery stores to open in what are now food desert communities. There is a responsibility to overcome these negative attitudes, and we also must address how the government can work together with more localized community groups. We are on our way to redesigning the current governmental programs to help promote and encourage healthy habits by making the healthy choice be the affordable choice. Already, devices are in place in the Supplemental Nutrition Assistance Program (SNAP) that double the monetary amount of assistance at farmer's markets, where shoppers can buy healthy produce. Here, the social contract is reinforced through farmer's market vendors committing to honor a buyer's government assistance benefits, thereby giving community members the ability to make healthy choices.

Community engagement is sometimes a hurdle to undertaking meaningful action. Often, conversations around our responsibilities to conservation or environmental concerns can be especially driven down to a very individual level. For example, when talking about conserving water or energy, the dialogue focuses on coaching people to turn off their faucets, unplug unused appliances, or drive less, which are all very individualized responsibilities. The moderator of the second morning panel focusing on the Great Lakes, Susan Heffernan of WBEZ Chicago, asked the panelists about these kinds of small-scale interventions and how this discourse may disempower people from wanting to engage in these conversations, whether it be from feelings of guilt for not engaging in these measures and feeling wasteful, or because they do not feel their small efforts alone can make a difference. We must involve the general public in broader policy conversations that have the potential to create a larger paradigm shift; such conversations will help community members recognize how their actions can have a larger impact. Governments at all scales will benefit from engaging residents and working together on policy solutions.

Education is crucial in facilitating the public engagement that has historically driven broad public support. Educating people about the condition of the Great Lakes depends on the public having access to the informative research that is being done. David Ullrich, executive director of the Great Lakes and St. Lawrence Cities Initiative, discussed U.S. and Canadian reports examining how the health of the Great Lakes can be expressed through a complex series of indicators, and boiled down to "the few [key indicators] that tell us the most." Being able to simplify the most important elements for a healthy ecosystem will allow for a broader public understanding of the problems facing the Great Lakes. With greater understanding of the state of the Great Lakes comes a greater ability for the public to engage in the social contract and for all of us to bring about broader policy changes that affect the entire region. The ecosystem of the Great Lakes covers an immense amount of land and encompasses many jurisdictions. The region is full of small governments dealing with each piece of the ecosystem individually. The Clean Water Act (CWA) is a federally enacted policy that helped to bring about a broader conversation about our resources. Those in the Great Lakes region enjoy as a right what Henderson describes as "the ability to have access to this amazing commons for personal appropriation," and they can misjudge their role in the shared interests of the entire ecosystem. It will become increasingly critical to govern and manage this region as "a conjoined joined ecosystem where the health of waters in pristine trout streams going into Lake Superior are of interest to the people in Toledo." Because the entire region is connected, any policy implementations will be felt in all Great Lakes cities. The social contract must dictate how our next policy considerations for the region must also consider the importance of coordinating laws and practices across jurisdictions for the sake of each individual community's shared interest in the Great Lakes.

Henderson also reiterated how large-scale action can be difficult because of "people sorting themselves into particular small communities of discourse" where the broader conversation can be polarizing to certain communities, which threatens the social contract. For example, the use of the phrase "climate change" resonates differently in different communities, which makes addressing the issue challenging. When the United States passed the Clean Air Act and the Clean Water Act in 1963 and 1972, respectively, environmental health was a bipartisan national issue. However, our society's discourse today is so fragmented and polarized that even the well-being of our environment is disputed, which compromises the social contract.

This unfortunate polarization means that an environmental frame will not always resonate with an audience, and we must find ways to reach people with stories that matter to them. Sometimes, environmental issues must be described in terms of other economic or cultural values. Suzanne Malec-McKenna, executive director of Chicago Wilderness, explained that discussions about climate may fall on deaf ears in some audiences, so she must instead change the conversation and discuss the benefits of reduced flooding, or consistent returns on investment for environmentally friendly infrastructure. Diversifying the conversations about these issues will help more people feel compelled to act. Ullrich also mentioned disasters like wildfires and flooding that have devastating environmental consequences. However, some people need monetary values to be placed on these disasters, through loss of property value, or lives lost, in order to fully appreciate the destruction caused by these events.

Malec-McKenna also emphasized the importance of connecting these conversations back to a health framework. In Lake County, for example, a trend has emerged of physicians writing "nature scripts": patients with cardiac, respiratory, or diabetic conditions who could benefit from engaging with their natural surrounding are being given "prescriptions" to take walks in nature. Highlighting the health benefits to engaging with their natural surroundings can have mass appeal to diverse communities and help promote a healthy region.

## OUR RESPONSIBILITY TO THE SOCIAL CONTRACT

The Great Lakes region plays a huge role in the United States as a water resource, but our region is also a crossroads for energy transportation. Energy resources move through, and on, the Great Lakes by pipelines, trains, and ships. These resources are critical commodities but are also potentially dangerous to a region's ecology. Protecting public health and the environment to fill our energy needs relies on the wise management of crude oil, natural gas, and coal traveling through the region. With the shift from using Middle

Eastern to using North American oil came an exponential increase in the use of railways to transport the crude oil to the refineries through the Great Lakes region. The safety measures in place (including the standards for tanks, rail braking systems, volatility levels of the crude oil, and oversight of operators and employees) were not initially sufficient to safely manage this huge volume of oil being transported through the region. Even additional U.S. and Canadian regulations were still sometimes insufficient to prevent disaster in the Great Lakes region and beyond. Ullrich refers to the 2013 derailment of a freight train carrying crude oil through Lac-Mégantic in Québec that virtually demolished the downtown area after the cars exploded, resulting in forty-seven deaths, and the 2010 pipeline break in Kalamazoo, Michigan, operated by Enbridge that resulted in the largest inland oil spill in U.S. history. The entire Great Lakes region will continue to face the dangers associated with oil transport through rail and through pipelines as safety regulations and policies evolve. Tighter regulations and better enforcement will be necessary to ensure the safety of the region. All communities of the Great Lakes and beyond will depend on the social contract and being able to rely on those charged with transporting the oil to do so responsibly.

Both U.S. and Canadian federal governments have a responsibility in enacting laws and programs to ensure the safe transport of oil through the Great Lakes region. There are inconsistent requirements through the multiple jurisdictions that are impacted by this industry, and Ullrich emphasized the need for "harmonization of requirements between the U.S. and Canada." It is not feasible for the mayor of a single municipality in the Great Lakes region to get any satisfaction dealing directly with a major oil corporation like Enbridge, so communities should be able to rely on their federal government to speak up for them.

Pipelines transporting crude oil require both intense pressure and heat. Current regulations for pipelines are inadequate because they do not reflect these technical needs and are not capable of managing different types of oil transport, such as rail. In the event of a spill, crude oil will behave differently in the environment depending on what type of crude it is, and responses to these disasters depend on having management tools and regulations in place that can respond appropriately. However, discussion too often revolves around *reactive* strategies, rather than setting proactive goals that the Clean Water Act and Clean Air Act meant to control. There is a need to strengthen the government's role to better enforce these regulations so they actually can fulfill their role of protecting the environment.

Another key measure in the broader context will be to acknowledge the reality of climate change. By doing this, we can start to more critically analyze our reliance on fossil fuels and realize the importance of finding alternative energy sources. Before we can reach this stage however, we must rely on effectively regulating the industry practices.

Many businesses, however, may not agree that regulations are the solution to ensuring safety. Heffernan speculates that Enbridge's response would be that increased regulation would only further impede business, and that they are employing all possible safety measures to fulfill their role to society by providing people with the energy they need. Malec-McKenna offered that demonstrating to companies how their investments in more socially conscious practices can positively impact their bottom lines may be more effective in making them more mindful of their social impacts on the region. It is inevitable that businesses will always be concerned with their shareholders and the economic impacts of their policy making. Working with this reality could more effectively encourage more private investments to diversify the funding sources for the region. Ullrich agreed with Malec-McKenna's characterization, noting that companies need to take seriously consumer and social pressures. This helps to link everyone into the social contract where all parties are able to benefit.

There is also work being done to help utility companies make money through greater efficiency, rather than through selling more electricity to customers. Proper regulations and enforcement of regulations will allow us to incentivize companies to increase efficiency and still be able to be profitable. Programs like Retrofit Chicago are creating jobs and reducing operating costs for buildings through green practices, and they are also making positive impacts in addressing climate change.

Malec-McKenna agreed that the broader public conversation could be better facilitated not only through greater awareness of the issues with the ecosystem but also through discussions about the economic impact of conserving our natural resources. It is sometimes difficult for this argument to resonate with the people of the Great Lakes because these resources come cheap in this region. Both water and energy resources in the Great Lakes region are less costly compared to elsewhere in the United States. She also points out that the cost of waste removal in the region is only a quarter of what residents pay in coastal cities like San Francisco. Economic incentives resonate with the public differently than the moral arguments for conservation, and by translating the value of conservation efforts into nature economics we can better engage different populations throughout the region. Acknowledging the diversity of the broader population and connecting with local values will also help empower communities to take action for the sake of the entire region.

As we continue to consider the elements of a social contract moving forward, we must bear in mind the interconnectedness of health, energy, and the environment. Good health and wellness stem from a healthy environment, which relies on responsible energy consumption. All actors in society—governments, businesses, and individuals—have roles to play in supporting the health and safety of the public, as well as of the environment. Only through working together and acknowledging both the shared interests, as well as core interests of each sector, can we empower each other and successfully fulfill the social contract. Recognition of those institutions whose central design is to promote our health, safety, and the environment, is critical to encouraging public debate and discourse, and therefore critical to progress. As Henry Henderson notes, "We need to be focusing on structures that are supportive, and cultivate the safety and dignity of people and communities."

# Contributors

**ALBA ALEXANDER** is visiting associate professor of political science at the University of Illinois at Chicago. Her research interests include taxation, urban politics, and the welfare state. Her articles have appeared in such journals as *Congress and the Presidency, International Journal of Urban and Regional Research, Harvard International Review,* and *Soziale Welte.* She is the author of *Playing Fair: The Politics of Taxation in the US* (forthcoming) and is coeditor with Dennis Judd and Evan McKenzie of *Reconstituting the Local State* (forthcoming).

**MEGAN HOUSTON** is a master's degree candidate in the College of Urban Planning and Public Affairs at the University of Illinois at Chicago.

**DENNIS R. JUDD** is department head and professor in the Department of Political Science at the University of Illinois at Chicago. His writings include the textbook *City Politics: Private Power and Public Policy* (2014, 9th ed.) and pioneering research on urban tourism. As part of this continuing research program he has coedited *The Tourist City* (with Susan S. Fainstein, 1999), *Cities and Visitors: Regulating Cities, Markets, and City Space* (with Lily M. Hoffman and Susan S. Fainstein, 2004), and *The City, Revisited: Urban Theory from Chicago, Los Angeles, and New York* (with Dick Simpson, 2011). He is coauthor of *Mayor Richard M. Daley and the Rise of Chicago's City of Spectacle* (with Costas Spirou, forthcoming).

**CYNTHIA KLEIN-BANAI** is associate chancellor for sustainability at the University of Illinois at Chicago (UIC), an office that she founded. Prior to her current position, she was assistant director for chemical safety in the Environmental Health and Safety Office at UIC. There she oversaw environmental compliance, hazardous waste management, the laboratory safety program, and chemical safety training. She has also worked as an environmental consultant. Her university career started at the University of Illinois at Urbana-Champaign Division of Environmental Health and Safety, where she studied pollution prevention in laboratories.

**WILLIAM C. KLING** is an attorney and public-policy expert with over twenty-five years' experience in the public and nonprofit sectors. He currently has an appointment at University of Illinois Chicago School of Public Health, Health Policy and Administration Division, and serves as a policy research specialist for UIC and University of Illinois Urbana-Champaign, as well as several other governmental and nongovernmental organizations. Kling has been engaged in public policy work concerning sustainability, water resource management, the 2007 Farm Bill, and other community-based capacity building initiatives. His work has been funded by the W. K. Kellogg Foundation, the Robert Woods Johnson Foundation, the Otho A. Sprague Memorial Institute, and the Northeast Midwest Institute, among other institutions. Dr. Kling is active in many professional development and community activities, including serving on the boards of the South Cook Healthcare Consortium, the Plant Chicago, and Econ Illinois. He speaks and writes regularly on a variety of topics.

**HOWARD A. LEARNER** is a public interest attorney who serves as the president and executive director of the Environmental Law & Policy Center, the Midwest's premier public-interest environmental legal advocacy and eco-business innovation organization, and among the nation's leaders in those fields. He is also an adjunct professor at the University of Michigan Law School and at Northwestern University Law School, where he teaches advanced seminars in energy and environmental law, climate change policy, and sustainable development law. Learner received his JD from Harvard Law School (1980) and BA from the University of Michigan (1976).

**DAVID A. MCDONALD** is professor of global development studies at Queen's University, Canada. He is also codirector of the Municipal Services Project, a research initiative exploring alternatives to the privatization of service provision in electricity, health, water, and sanitation in Africa, Asia, and Latin America. His previous works include *Rethinking Corporatization and Public*

*Services in the Global South* (2014) and *World City Syndrome: Neoliberalism and Inequality in Cape Town* (2008).

**DAVID C. PERRY** is a professor of Urban Planning and Policy in the College of Urban Planning and Public Affairs at the University of Illinois at Chicago (UIC). He served as director of the Great Cities Institute at UIC and the associate chancellor for the university's Great Cities Commitment. He is now senior fellow at GCI. Perry is the author or editor of twelve books and contributes journalistic pieces to, for example, the *New York Times*, the *Nation*, and *Metropolis* magazine. His service includes numerous community partners and having served on national and local public boards and commissions, including Chicago's Zoning Reform Commission, the Urban Land Institute's National Public Infrastructure Committee, the Chicago Council on Global Affairs, the Rudy Bruner National Award Selection Committee, the National Task Force on Anchor Institutions, and the Strengthening Communities Strand of the Coalition of Urban Serving Universities of the Association of Public Land Grant Universities.

**EMILY STIEHL** is a clinical assistant professor of health policy and administration in the University of Illinois at Chicago School of Public Health. Her research examines employee outcomes (e.g., job attachment and extra-role behaviors at work) among the working poor, and the impact of poverty on work attitudes and behaviors. In addition to looking at the effects of poverty on individual workers, her research also considers how organizations could ameliorate the situation of the working poor in practice. Much of her research has focused on certified nursing assistants.

**ANTHONY TOWNSEND** is senior research scientist at New York University's Rudin Center for Transportation Policy and Management, where he supervises research on the impact of information and communication technologies on mobility, land use, and transportation planning. He is the author of *Smart Cities: Big Data, Civic Hackers, and the Quest for a New Utopia* (2013). His writing and research have appeared in *Scientific American, Stanford Social Innovation Review*, and *Cairo Review of Global Affairs*. He is frequently quoted in technology and business publications and broadcasts, including the *New York Times*, the *Economist*, NPR, *BusinessWeek*, and *Time*.

**NATALIA VILLAMIZAR-DUARTE** is a doctoral student in the College of Urban Planning and Public Affairs, University of Illinois at Chicago.

**MOIRA ZELLNER** is associate professor in the College of Urban Planning and Public Affairs at the University of Illinois at Chicago. She has served primary investigator and coinvestigator for interdisciplinary projects studying how specific policy, technological, and behavioral changes can effectively address a range of complex environmental problems, where interaction effects make responsibilities and burdens unclear. Her research also examines the value of complexity-based modeling for participatory policy exploration and social learning with stakeholders. Moira teaches a variety of workshops on complexity-based modeling of socio-ecological systems, for training of both scientists and decision makers.

**THE URBAN AGENDA**

Metropolitan Resilience in a Time of Economic Turmoil
*Edited by Michael A. Pagano*

Technology and the Resilience of Metropolitan Regions
*Edited by Michael A. Pagano*

The Return of the Neighborhood as an Urban Strategy
*Edited by Michael A. Pagano*

Remaking the Urban Social Contract: Health, Energy, and the Environment
*Edited by Michael A. Pagano*